Essential Oils and Aromatherapy

Discover the Ancient Powerful Remedy

By Jason Bright

Copyright © 2019 by Jason Bright

Table of Contents

Introduction

Today's world is a world aimed at making everything simple, light and easy; including healing. You have a headache, take some Tylenol. If you don't have at home, you could walk into a store and get it. It's that simple. Yet, treating headaches or any other kind of ailment wasn't so simple in ancient times. It required in-depth knowledge of the wonders of plant life as well as some expertise in making the tinctures and potions that could actually work.

The technology available to ancient civilizations could not enable them to extract and combine the chemical compounds needed to create the kind of pharmaceuticals we have, both in quantity and size. In spite of this, they tapped into the raw elements of plant life itself. These ancients thrived on herbalism.

Archeological evidence has shown that humans had begun utilizing plants for their medicine and healing since the Paleolithic age. Healing plant recipes from Egypt, Greece, India, and China have been discovered in extensive medical records that documented about 3,000 years ago. It would appear that these civilizations had discovered and harnessed the healing powers of plants.

From ancient Egyptian texts, garlic, castor bean, cannabis, and juniper were the predominant plants used for healing. The Chinese also used hemp, Ephedra, and Chaulmogra mainly for skin diseases, breathing and digestion problems. Rosemary, ginger, lemongrass, thyme, and Chamomile are some of the plants that were used for healing in those times.

The usage of these plants was also something that was very unique. Some of these plants were dried and then preserved for future use. Some were boiled in water while the patient drank the plant-infused water. Some plants were also made into a paste and rubbed on wounds and parts of the body that needed healing, like, swollen parts and burn injuries.

Back then, it was relatively easy to gain access to the natural medicine they used. Let us not forget that natural medicine encompasses the herbs to use, as well as, the process and dosage of use. This knowledge was available to many members of society who had gained the knowledge through oral tradition and documented remedies.

As the centuries progressed, the oral tradition began to diminish. Then, there arose a group of individuals who had managed to preserve the knowledge they had. They were called physicians. These people began to seek out more plants and more ways to make healing faster and better. They conducted various experiments. They created diverse herbal mixtures. They delved into extensive studies of the human body.

In spite of the impressive work these physicians did, they had one great problem. The herbal mixtures they made could not last long enough. In times of emergency, they would need to begin the lengthy and stressful process of preparing their mixtures. Most times, both patients and healers didn't have the luxury of time. Yet, they needed to these mixtures. The number of people interested in the art of healing started to dwindle. It was then that physicians came up with a solution to their problems. They discovered that oils had the capacity to absorb the compounds of plants that facilitate healing. Then, they were set on discovering how to combine the extracts of the plants with oils. It was then that the concept of what we now know as essential oils were birthed. The problem of shortage and preservation had been dealt with.

As physicians began to uncover different ways of integrating plant extracts with oil, there was an increase in the variety of essential oils. According to findings, Ibn al-Baitar was the first physician to begin and extensive work on essential oils. His work, along with that of his colleagues, led to the creation of oils like lavender oil, basil oil, bay oil, cedar oil, citron oil, moringa oil, ginger oil amongst others.

What is most astonishing is that studies have shown that these oils were very effective; sometimes even more effective than the drugs we now have. Not only did they serve as healing agents, but they also had very few side effects. Even though Western science has placed essential oils into the category of alternative medicine, the truth still remains that essential oils are just as effective as modern pharmaceuticals are.

Chapter One

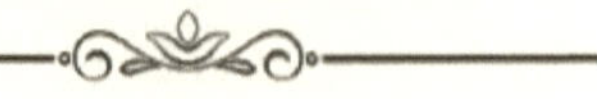

What Are Essential Oils

Essential oil is a term that is very prominent in the world of alternative medicine. The name appears so lyrical; *essential oils.* Yet, few people are actually aware of what these oils are.

Essential oils are condensed chemical compounds that have been gathered from plant extracts. In simple words, essential oils are plant extracts that encapsulate the essence of the plant itself. These extracts are the life juices of the plants that are acquired by cold pressing, distillation (which is basically, steaming the plants till the essence is obtained) and other ways which will be disclosed subsequently.

In the process of making essential oils, each and every part of the plant is used. The seeds, the roots, the leaves, the steam are very vital in the process of making essential oils. This is to ensure that all of the healing properties of the plant are gotten. Once the process is done, the essential oil is named after the plant it was made from.

The most significant feature of essential oils is that they are extremely volatile. This means that their form can change from a solid state to liquid and to a gaseous state. This entire change can occur even when the temperature is normal. Indeed, this quality is what makes it easy for the scent of the oil to make its way to the nostrils and the senses and perform the appropriate function it needs to do.

Essential oils can be used in various ways. Essential oils can be inhaled (in fact, aromatherapists and essential oil experts have stated that this is the best way to use essential oils). Essential oils can also be used on the skin. It depends on whatever function you need it to perform. However, you must be sure to find out that the oils are safe enough to be used on the skin. You must also check if you have a skin that is too sensitive for essential oils to be used on. Be aware that you can never ingest any type of essential oil without proper guidance from experts. To do so will be too expose yourself to various kinds of health complications and toxic poisoning. Due to the high concentration of natural compounds in essential oils, it is essential (pun intended) that the oils are diluted before use.

Although essential oils have been placed under the category of alternative medicine, they are just as effective as conventional drugs. They do the same work that these drugs do with none of the side effects that come with the drugs. Sometimes, essential oils even do a much better job than pharmaceuticals. Studies have shown that essential oils can eradicate a kind of Lyme bacteria. Astonishingly, the oils can kill the bacteria even faster than antibiotics can. Essential oils can cure headaches and insomnia, relieve stress and anxiety and reduce depression. They also help in treating various skin diseases such as acne, eczema and all others.

One common misconception is that essential oils and fragrance oils are the same. Essential oils are pure plant extracts that are primarily meant for healing. Fragrance or perfume oils, on the other hand, are oils that have fragrances of certain sweet-smelling plants. The fragrances are mixed with synthetic oils for quantity and preservation. In aromatherapy, fragrance oils are considered helpful. Yet, when it comes to quality and effectiveness, essential oils rank higher than fragrance oils. So, take care to never assume that perfume oils can be substituted for essential oils.

In essence, the condensed extracts of a certain plant are what we call essential oil. We now know what makes essential oils. We know what they can do. Nonetheless, we need to ask ourselves why these plants are called essential oils, instead of some other fancy name.

Essential oils are the objects of delight. They have wonderful scents. They heal just as conventional drugs do and they do not have fatal side effects. Yet, one must wonder why these plant extracts are called essential oils. There could have been any other name for the extracts. Why "essential oils"?

Alchemists stumbled upon essential oils as they searched for another element to be added to water, fire, air, and earth. After it was first discovered that plants had healing properties that could be extracted, deciding the nature of these extracts was very difficult. After all, one could obtain the properties of a plant by soaking the leaves in hot water. What was so different about this process? After much contemplation, the alchemists back then decided to name these oils, *essential oils*.

First, the oils were the life juices gathered from the entire plant- not just the leaves or the roots. The core of the plant is taken by distillation, maceration or mechanical pressing. This core is then condensed into a form that is highly volatile.

Secondly, the oils were christened *essential oils* because the alchemists and physicians of old believed that the oils signified the real essence of flavor and odor. Remember, essential oils are some of the few healing substances that function effectively via smell-regardless of the type or kind. The essential oils still retain the flavor of the plant, as well. So, the name essential oils seemed like a wonderful option.

One other reason essential oils are named as such lies in the process of its retrieval. In the Renaissance period, distillation became the best way to get the "pure" elements that are encased by non-volatile and impure items. Distillation became a means of unearthing the vital things from irrelevant things. Back then, distillation was the most popular way to obtain oils. So, the process itself ensured that the oils were still being tagged "essential".

Surprisingly, essential oils are not oily. The oils are not just soluble in water. Again, the tag "oil" can be traced to the time of its discovery. In those times, anything that could not be dissolved in water was termed an oil. Essential oils can be dissolved in vegetable oils, fatty acids, amongst other items in the oil and fats category. Yet, this singular feature prompted the alchemists to call the extracts "oils" and the tag has stuck ever since.

Over time, the meaning of the word "essence" expanded to mean: fragrance, flavor. This semantic broadening also affected the meaning of essential oils. Essential oils came to be referred to as such because of how easy it was to make essences for perfumes and food flavors. Like it was stated earlier, essential oils are soluble in anything apart from water. While making fragrances, flavorings, disinfectants, and other items, the oils are dissolved in alcohol to sharpen and heighten their effects. The change in the use of the essential oils also reinforced its name and significance.

As the discipline of botany became more advanced and concrete, essential oils began to be called other names. Sometimes, they are called volatile oils. "Volatile" refers to the oils' level of volatility. Essential oils can change from solid to gaseous at room temperature. In science- chemistry, specifically- this process is called volatility. Essential oils are also known as ethereal oils. Also, this is in line with the volatile nature of the oils. Amongst other things, "ethereal" means " exceeding light or airy in form". It is very easy for essential oils to dissipate into the air. So, "ethereal oils" is also a perfect name for the plant extracts.

Discovering the origin behind the name "essential oil" is not just to satisfy another curiosity about essential oils. It is a means of understanding essential oils as a whole. It is also an attempt to grasp how these oils are gotten. More importantly, it is a trip down the history of essential oils. This layer of essential oils has been dealt with. Yet, what is left to know about essential oils is yet to be fully uncovered.

Chapter Two

Aromatherapy

Every minute we spend in our environment leaves an impression on us both mentally and physically and it doesn't matter if what we feel is pleasant or not. Our sensual experiences are able to control our mood, movement, hormones, feeling, thinking, resistance to illness and metabolism. We are wired to lean towards and place ourselves around a natural environment whenever we feel stressed because we acknowledge that natural elements are able to restore us to a complete mental and physical state.

Humans started using fragrant flowers, resins, plants, woods during the time of the Neanderthals who used aromatic flowers and herbs to bury their dead.

The ancient Egyptians, Arabs, and Romans had several uses for scents including skincare, air purification, the healing of wounds and embalmment.

Some people even believed that essential oils were more precious than gold and this prompted grave robbers to raid King Tutankhamun's tomb in search of it.

Some other cultures used fragrant flowers in their religious worship practices, perfumes, antiseptic and antibiotic.

In the early 20th century, medicinal practices included aromas. A French perfumer and chemist, Rene Maurice Gattefosse found out that applying lavender oil to a burn on his hand helped it heal very fast. He noticed the oil was therapeutic while also being aromatic and that birthed the term Aromatherapy.

Wholistic aromatherapists have been able to use oils as therapy by creating unique blends based on individual problems. Prescriptions are made for individuals to soothe their mind body and spirit depending on their scent choices and symptoms.

When we perceive a pleasant smell, it triggers relaxation, helps us to breathe and keeps us away from the physical and emotional effects of stress and scents extracted from nature are most effective in improving our general well-being both mentally, physically, emotionally and spiritually.

The modern life we live disconnects us from nature but we are connected to nature by the fragrant essential oils extracted from plants and their parts.

Basically, the therapeutic fragrances we smell in nature are all gotten from essential oils.

Benefits of Aromatherapy

Aromatherapy and essential oils do not hold the cure for all illnesses but help in balancing emotions. This is what we should remember when we hear the word "aromatherapy".

The human body has about 400 types of scent receptors. It is able to detect several different smells and the scent receptors are more than the number of receptors the body has for other senses.

People are able to differentiate between smells that they perceive even though they may not have the words to describe them. Memories that are triggered by scents are often the ones that move us the most.

When we perceive some scents, we are energized and these scenes can bring us to a balanced state if we are being overstimulated.

All essential oils do not benefit all users in the same exact way. A person's reaction to a scent can be affected by the past memories attached to it.

For instance, Rose oil is known to help people who are grieving. The scent may do the opposite and trigger a negative experience for someone if, say, the smell triggers memories of an abusive relative who may have worn a rose-scented perfume. However, if the relative was kind, the scent will produce a positive response and will be effective as a stress relief for that individual.

In aromatherapy, a person should not be forced to use a scent that they do not have any natural attraction to even if it is prescribed for their emotional issue.

This is why Marguerite Maury came up with an Individual Prescription Technique in the 1950s. The biochemist majored in holistic aromatherapy and innovated a special massage technique to apply essential oils. Her patients were prescribed different oils based on their emotional and physical development.

The oils form a unique blend that tends to cater to the individual's mind, spirit and body because Holistic aromatherapy blends do not use one scent for all cases. The blends are created by a qualified practitioner for individuals depending on their symptoms and scent preferences.

How Essential Oils Get Into The Body

Essential oils enter the body system in three ways: inhalation, dermal absorption, and oral ingestion.

Using the ingestion method is not so safe unless it is done with prescription and under the supervision of a qualified medical practitioner.

Essential oils are most often produced for external use and this makes inhalation the most potent way of experiencing how therapeutic essential oils are.

1. Dermal Absorption

When essential oils are applied on the skin, the amount of oil that's absorbed depends on some conditions. When the essential oil is less viscous or applied over more skin area or applied on unclogged skin, a large amount of it will be absorbed. Some parts of the body with thinner skin also make it easy to absorb the oils like the soles of the feet, behind the ears, scalp, palms of hands, inside of wrists and armpits.

2. Oral Ingestion

This is actually the least effective way to use essential oil. This is because the oil gets to go through the slower digestive tract and pass several organs before eventually reaching the bloodstream.

Before it gets to the bloodstream, the chemical composition will be altered in the organs before the body finally gets rid of it.

3. Direct inhalation

Apart from stimulating the brain to trigger a reaction, natural essential oils can be inhaled into the lungs to release their chemical properties and provide therapeutic benefits.

For instance, you can ease congestion by diffusing eucalyptus essential oil.

Direct inhalation is simply breathing in the scent of essential oil. There are some methods to do it.

1. Breathe in the scent directly from an open essential oil bottle.

2. Drop some oil or a blend of oils on your hands, rub your hands and cup them around your nose and mouth and inhale.

However, remember to dilute when necessary to prevent skin irritation.

3. Drop some oil or a blend of oils on a piece of fabric or tissue, bring it close to the face and breathe in.

4. You can also diffuse essential oils with a spray bottle. Mix some oil with water or alcohol and spray in the air, on the body or other surfaces.

5. Diffusing the essential oils in a room is another popular method of aromatherapy. With a diffuser, the essential oil evaporates into the surroundings. This can help to change your mood by helping you relax or stimulate the mind. Diffusion can even help to get rid of airborne pathogens and heal a respiratory illness.

These are some of the ways you can diffuse essential oils:

- ❖ Diffuse a mix of cinnamon, clove, rosemary, eucalyptus, orange and lemon oils to clean the air.
- ❖ Diffuse peppermint to boost energy.
- ❖ Diffuse lavender to relieve stress and bring relief for a headache.

There are four types of diffusers:

1. Vaporizing: When using this diffuser, water is added to the essential oil and then the oil and water particles are spread into the air using ultrasonic waves. Vaporizing diffusers often make no sounds and which is why they are often chosen by yoga instructors, therapists and every other person who wants a peaceful environment.

2. Atomizing: This kind of diffuser does not need water. The essential oil bottle is connected so that only pure vapor is diffused and this is very potent and therapeutic.

3. Fan or evaporative: This kind of diffuser can be gotten at a low cost and is often used for smaller areas. A pad or filter is filled with essential oils and a fan blows air through it. The air that comes through the pad makes the oils to evaporate faster than it would in other diffusers.

4. Heat: Heat diffusers are similar to the evaporative diffusers because they allow the essential oils to fast. They diffuse through heat and not by blowing any air.

Topical Use Of Essential Oils

Essential oils are absorbed directly from the skin into the bloodstream because they are fat-soluble. Oftentimes, carrier oil is used to apply essential oil to the skin. But a "neat" application is when the oil is applied without needing a carrier oil. A neat application is often used when applying oils to the soles of the feet.

It is even a popular site for oil application for many reasons:

- ❖ Less irritation: There is a lower chance of skin irritation when oils are applied to the soles of the feet. This is because the skin around there has little sensitivity compared to the skin on other body parts.

- ❖ No sebum: The only sites on the body that do not have sebaceous glands are the soles of the feet and the palm of the hands. Sebum is the oily substance that acts as a lubricant and keeps the skin waterproof. Because they are unable to secrete sebum, they easily absorb oil.

- ❖ Bypass the liver: Oils applied to the soles of the feet bypass the liver and do not settle there. They are not processed by the liver rather they travel through the lower bronchial capillaries through the circulatory system and reach the body unprocessed.

The other key places where essential oils can be applied include the abdomen, behind the ears, along the spine, temples and upper back. Avoid sensitive areas like the inner ears, open skin, genitals, and eyes, during application.

For topical application, essential oils are most often used together with a carrier oil. The carrier oil dilutes the essential oil and also stops it from evaporating easily thereby reducing the possibility of having a skin reaction.

The top carrier oils include jojoba oil, pomegranate seed oil, coconut oil, avocado oil, almond oil, olive oil, and grapeseed oil.

Jojoba oil: It helps to maintain balance in both oily and very dry skin. It is often used with lavender, geranium, and tea tree oil.

Coconut oil: This all-purpose oil is the best choice for personal care products, and apart from its topical use with essential oils, it is a necessary ingredient in making deodorants, lotions, and toothpaste.

Shea butter: This carrier oil is often best as a moisturizer for aged and very dry skin.

Magnesium oil: It is often mixed with Roman chamomile and lavender to improve sleep and reduce stress.

Arnica oil: It is the best option for treating pain, inflammation, and bruises.

Argan oil: It provides anti-aging effects and helps to tighten and firm skin. It boosts skin tone when combined with myrrh, geranium, and frankincense.

Other useful carrier oils include hemp, rosehip, Sea buckthorn, black cumin, and apricot.

When applying essential oils topically, be mindful of the dose. Consider the age and size of the individual. Smaller amounts of oil are required for young and small people.

The safest method is to start the application with a small amount and if necessary apply again after 20 minutes.

You can dilute the essential oil and carrier oil with this ratio:

For Infants

1 drop of essential oil should be mixed with 1 tablespoon carrier oil.

For children

1 to 2 drops of essential oil should be mixed with 1 teaspoon carrier oil.

For Adults

3 to 6 drops of essential oil should be mixed with 1 teaspoon carrier oil.

After diluting, rub the oils together with your fingers and palm then apply on the area of concern in circular, calm massage movements.

Other topical uses include

1. Baths

Using essential oils in bath water is a combination of topical and aromatic applications. To help the oil disperse properly in the water, put 5 to 15 drops of essential oil on Epsom salts or bath salts. The oils will spread when they dissolve in the water. This method helps to enhance circulation, open the airways, improve sleep, soothe skin, calm sore muscles and relax the body. An aromatherapy bath is more effective with oils like lavender and eucalyptus.

2. Compresses

The essential oils are easily absorbed when a warm compress is used.

Create a mixture with 10 drops of essential oil for every 4 ounces of water. Soak a cloth in the mixture and rub it on aches, pains, bruises, and infections.

3. Salves

This is an ointment made to calm the body's surface. Prepare a salve with 15 drops of essential oil and 1 ounce of carrier oil. Store it in a metal or glass container. Salves are used on sore muscles, cuts, and scrapes.

4. Personal care

Many home items are made from essential oils like deodorant, shampoo, toothpaste, lip balm, face wash, body lotion, shampoo, perfume, and cologne.

Chapter Three

Safety and Precautions

Are essential oils safe to use?

Essential oils have become the most sought after products in the wellness industry. Apparently, the industry is now worth 12 billion dollars. Yet, the ever-increasing popularity of the oils seemed to fuel the reservations people have about their safety. People keep asking, "Are essential oils really safe to use?" In the surge of demand for alternative medical products, skeptics are also beginning to fuel the worries and concerns about the safety of the users of these essential oils.

Numerous dermatologists and aromatherapists, alongside medical experts, have confirmed that essential oils are very safe to use. Nonetheless, they need the right use, proper prescription, and accurate dosage- just like conventional drugs. Apart from the directives and recommendation given by experts, there are other things to consider when assessing how safe a certain essential oil is- especially if you are going to use it personally. These factors include age, existing health conditions, and medical history, means of usage, manner of usage, duration and dosage.

Age

There are some oils that must never be used for people of certain ages. These oils might end up being too potent for the individuals' immune system. For instance, peppermint oil should not be used for children as it can affect their breathing. The same thing applies to old people. Lavender oil could also deter body growth in male teenagers. So, age can be what determines how safe it is for you to use essential oil. There are some oils that must not be used around or on children. These might pose severe health challenges for the children. The essential oils should only be used on the children if-and only if-they are recommended by a specialist. Such oils include peppermint, eucalyptus, fennel, rosemary, verbena, and Wintergreen.

Manner of usage

It has been reiterated that essential oils should only be inhaled or used on the skin. Essential oils are not to be used internally or in any areas of the mucous membranes. Places like the vagina, mouth, and eyes should not come in contact with essential oils for any reason.

There is one other thing that should be done before using any essential oil on your skin. You must find out if your skin will react to the oil. This process is called the patch test. Here is how it goes: First, you rub little essential oil on a small area on your arm. Then, you cover that part you have applied the oil on with a Band-Aid. After a few hours, take off the Band-Aid. If the area is red and itchy or the area has a rash, then you will know that that oil is not good for your skin. In that case, contact a dermatologist for more information. However, if that skin area is clear and free of any visible marks, then the oil is compatible with your skin. You are free to use it.

Purity

It was stated earlier that essential oils are highly concentrated- due to the number of plants it takes to get very small quantities of essential oil. This is why using them on the skin without diluting them is extremely dangerous. If you need to use essential oils on the skin, you must dilute them- not with water, of course, but with carrier oils (for example, olive oil and sesame oil). Generally, the concentration level of essential oils should be below 5 percent. Adding three drops of essential oil to an ounce of carrier oil does the trick. So, dilution is extremely important. You must also be wary of essential oils that have synthetic compounds in them. Some companies add synthetic chemicals to their essential oil products. This can also affect the safety of the usage of essential oils. Therefore, you must always get your oils from a company that is known for quality and authentic essential oil products.

To sum it all up, essential oils are as safe to use as any other type of medicine. It must be noted that each and every person that has had issues with essential oils faced their problems due to their failure to adhere to the precautionary principles and safety steps required to use essential oils. All in all, essential oils are safe to use in treating health conditions (physically, emotionally and psychologically).

Factors That Influence The Safety Of Essential Oils

We have explored the question of safety surrounding the use of essential oils. It was established that essential oils are indeed safe to use. Yet, there are certain factors that can determine if the oils will be safe for you to use or not. Here, we will be diving deeper into the factors that will determine your essential oil will work on you or if it will cause a seriously negative reaction.

Some of the factors that have been earlier discussed are; age, purity, and manner of use. In this chapter, the factors to be discussed include existing health conditions and medical history, skin sensitivity and phototoxicity, amongst others.

Existing Health Conditions and Medical History

Persons with certain health conditions are not supposed to use some essential oils. This is because there is no means of knowing how the body will respond to contact with the essential oil. In order to avoid unwarranted health complications, individuals with certain health conditions do not use some types of essential oils. For instance, asthma patients are advised to stay away from peppermint and eucalyptus oils. This is due to the pungent aroma that these oils have. To any other person, the oils are very good for curing headaches and staying alert. To asthma patients, on the other hand, it is a bane to their breathing and respiratory system. Cancer patients undergoing chemotherapy or medications to combat the cancer are always strongly advised to stay away from essential oils of any kind. The essential oils and conventional drugs could hinder each other from working on the patient's body. Worse still, the patient's body system could break down due to the high influx of chemicals in the body. So, one must seek to consider their health conditions and medical history before investing in any essential oil.

Skin Sensitivity

Essential oils do not often have negative effects on the skin- that is if it is used properly. Yet, some people's skin is extremely sensitive and requires the mildest contact with any type of skin product. For people like this, essential oils should not be applied to the skin. Inhalation is the best way for them to use essential oils– if the need arises. People with skin diseases and problems should seek the professional opinion of a dermatologist before using any type of essential oil.

Phototoxicity

Phototoxicity occurs when the skin becomes irritated after being exposed to the sun. This irritation occurs due to some previous skin application of a material that is not compatible with the skin. So, phototoxicity can take place when you step out into the sun immediately after you have just used certain types of essential oils. The essential oils that can induce phototoxicity are lemon oil, Angelica oil, lime oil and basically any essential oil obtained from citrus plants.

Time/Chemical Adulteration

The time range that a particular quantity of essential oil has been obtained from the plant(s) really matters. As time goes on, the chemical properties will begin to be altered. Even as the essential oil is exposed to heat and too much light, the changes will increase. Once these changes occur, the essential oils are no longer safe to use. Also, if the essential oils have been mixed with other synthetic chemicals by the company that produced the oils, then it is inadvisable to use such oil.

All these factors, along with the other factors mentioned earlier, are the crucial aspects that ensure that essential oil is safe for you to use.

In conclusion, essential oils are safe to use. Yet, the safety of their usage can easily be reversed if you do not stick with the rules guiding their use. Indeed, all it takes is following a few rules and you will be able to maximize the potentials of essential oils.

How To Know You're Getting High-Quality Oils

Determining the quality of products is a difficult task to do. It is even more tasking to do so for essential oils. The wellness industry is booming and teeming with success, high revenue, and profit-making. This certainly has its own advantages, but it comes with its downsides, as well. Many people want to cash in on the rapid growth of the sales of wellness products-, especially essential oils. This desperation will invariably lead to an increase in hoaxes and frauds in the essential oil business. Because of the nature of the product, it is very easy for crooks to put nonsense in a bottle and call it essential oil. This is the reason why you need to be aware of the qualities of authentic essential oil as well as the telltale signs of fake oils. Subsequently, we will be addressing the things to watch out for while buying quality essential oils.

Level of Purity

Before you buy your essential oil, you must make some inquiries and find out if the oil is 100 percent essential oil. Always make sure you are buying oils that do not have any kind of additives, synthetic chemicals or preservatives in them. Do not be deceived by any sales rep that claims that the essential oils need so and so chemical to make them work properly. Essential oils are pure oils that have been extracted from plants and nothing else. Any other chemical added to any essential oil has made it an adulterated oil.

Process of Extraction

The process through which essential oil is obtained affects its quality. Each type of extraction process has specific plants that are best suited to it. If any other type of extraction is used for such plants, the quality of the finished product will reduce. For instance, the lemon essential oil is best gotten through the cold pressing method. If the oil is gotten through solvent extraction, the oil will not be as efficient as the kind gotten through cold pressing. Hence, the process of extraction is a vital determinant of the quality of the finished product.

Price Range of Oil

The price of the essential oil you are about to buy really matters. Before buying any essential oil, you must find the cost of the same oil that other companies sell. If the price of the particular essential oil you want to buy is much cheaper than that of other brands, then you are probably buying a fake.

Packaging

This might appear absurd but how essential oil is packaged really matters. Essential oils are very volatile. Therefore, they must be placed in containers that cannot be perforated in any way. Glass bottles are the usual means of packaging. If the salesperson claims that the essential oil is pure, then it should be in a glass bottle. Only glass bottles have the capability of storing pure essential oils without any issue. Diluted essential oils can be stored in plastic and aluminum containers because they are no longer as potent as the pure essential oil. The bottle must also be sealed tight at the time of purchase. Every dealer knows that any leakage in the essential oil can lead to the loss of the entire product.

Provision of Botanical Name of the Plant

This is a simple professional touch that any company selling essential oils should add to their products. Even if the Latin name of the oil is not added to the label, it should be provided without hesitation when the customer asks for it. This simple phenomenon is what distinguishes essential oils of high quality from those that are not.

After all, if a person can go through the rigors of extracting an essential oil, the least they can do is to learn the botanical name of the essential oil.

All the things mentioned above are what you need to be aware of when checking out the quality of essential oils. There might be other factors but the ones mentioned above are very helpful in determining the quality of the essential oils you are interested in.

Precautions To Take When Using Essential Oils For Skin

Essential oils give you that skin you've been dreaming off but there are some precautions to observe while using it.

Even though essential oils are natural, you may get an allergic reaction from using it. Before you use any essential oil on your skin, do not forget to do a patch test.

Essential oils should not be used on the skin in their purest form. Make sure it's diluted with water, or carrier oil or your moisturizing lotion. They may cause negative reactions if used in its strong undiluted form.

Some essential oils are phototoxic (like lemon oil and others in the citrus family). This means that they react negatively when they are exposed to sunlight. The best time to use such oils is at night.

Pregnant women, children, and people who have epilepsy or high blood pressure should apply caution when using essential oils. It is advisable to not use any essential oil without regulation or permission from a doctor.

Be careful when storing essential oils because of their volatility. They are packaged in dark bottles to prevent sunlight and heat, so do well to keep them away from light and heat.

Also, do not expect essential oils to give you instant results. Exercise patience and keep to your routine religiously.

What Do You Do When You Have A Reaction?

Reaction to essential oils is a rare case but they also happen. If you are having a reaction to any essential oil that is topically applied, you may feel skin irritation or your skin may become more tender.

Before you use new oil, always do a patch test. Put one drop of oil on a tiny patch of skin on your forearm. If the oil is very hot or sensitive, dilute with five to ten drops of carrier oil before applying.

Notice how that small portion of skin reacts for an hour, even though any reaction will mostly show up in 10 minutes. If a reaction occurs, use fractionated coconut oil on it.

Be careful while using oils like Bergamot, lime, grapefruit, wild orange, lemon, tangerine and others belonging to the citrus family as they are photosensitive and will expose your skin to UV radiation and sunburn.

Do not get into direct sunlight for 12 hours after using the oil. If it will be inconvenient for you to do that, choose to diffuse them or use them internally or on a part of the skin that won't be exposed to light. Also, study essential oil blends carefully to ensure they do not include photosensitive oils.

Chapter Four

Oils As Ancient Medicine

In the beginning, plants were just plants-another slice of nature that was pleasing to the eyes. Sure, humans had begun to move from nomadic to communal. They had discovered that a plant could become a major source of food for them. Basically, plants were just for food and aesthetic purposes (and oxygen but they did not know this at the time). All this changed when Ancient Egyptians discovered that plants have certain elements that can be utilized for various purposes. Indeed, all the archeological and historical findings assert that Egyptians were the first to discover and use essential oils for medical treatment, adornment, and cosmetology as a whole. The oils were also used in the Egyptian embalming process.

The Greeks who also went to Egypt to learn also mastered the process of obtaining essential oils and the concept of aromatherapy, itself. Essential oils became so popular among the Greeks that the Greek physician, Hippocrates- who would later be known as the father of modern medicine-adopted essential oils as the core of his treatment. The Romans, too, were not left out, as they learned a lot about essential oils from the Greeks. The Romans would later weave essential oils into their lifestyle and culture by promoting essential oil-infused baths, oil fragrances, and hair products and interior decor based on the use of essential oils.

On the other side of the world, the Chinese and Indians had begun to delve deeper into the healing properties of plants alongside the process of retrieving it. Earlier on, the Chinese had discovered tea and its miraculous qualities. Still, they knew there had to be more to these plants than they knew. So, they kept on experimenting until they found their own variants of essential oils(ylang ylang oil, for instance). Eventually, these oils would become the pinnacle of Ayurvedic medicine – an ancient Indian medical system based on plants and herbs. The Chinese would also come to rely on them heavily for their medical treatment, as well.

The knowledge and use of essential oil spread wide and far from the Nile to palaces of the Roman emperors all the way to the exotic lands and nations in the East. Then, anarchy was set loose upon the West. The Roman Empire fell and religious subjugation became the order of the day. The Church shut down all the extensive work on essential oils. Instead, essential oils became the substitute for soap and water, as findings have shown- apparently, the Church was against bathing so the oils were used to reduce people's body odor.

Then again, the witch hunt that pervaded Europe from the 15th century to the 18th century did not help matters in any way. Anyone found with items (oils and tinctures included) that did not "align" with Christianity was tagged "occultic" and " spawn of the devil". That was a bad time for those qualities because that invariably meant such people would be burnt at the stakes. Naturally, the influx of essential oils reduced drastically until essential oils became an obsolete concept.

Interest in essential oils was not renewed until late in the 19th century. Charles Chamberland, a French microbiologist, was one of the pioneers in the research on essential oils and their antiseptic features. Many years later, one essential oil was uncovered as a total natural healing agent. The essential oil in question is lavender oil. This discovery was made by René Maurice Gattefossé, a French chemist and scholar. One day, he was conducting some experiments in the laboratory when a minor explosion occurred. The explosion got one of his hands burnt. Without thinking, he dunked his hand in the closest container of liquid he could find. Apparently, it was a tray of lavender oil. Incidentally, his hand got healed without any scar or infection. This propelled Gattefossé and many of his contemporaries to do extensive research on lavender oil and essential oils, as a whole. The rest, as they say, is history.

It would be prudent to assert that the interest in essential oils keeps increasing day after day. People are experiencing a reawakening in the use of natural healthcare products. People are tired of ingesting pharmaceuticals that would eventually lead to more complications in the long run. In the wake of this awareness, the next thing would be to know how these essential oils work.

Making Essential Oils

Essential oils are plant extracts (this has been said over and over again). How this process of extraction is done will be the focus of this chapter. There are various processes in extracting essential oils. They include distillation, solvent extraction, cold pressing, enfleurage, Carbon dioxide extraction, and Florasols. Subsequently, these processes will be discussed in full detail.

1. Distillation

Distillation is a process of separating the qualities of a mixture via selecting boiling and condensation. Distillation is the most popular process of extracting authentic essential oils. Distillation has various processes. Nonetheless, the one unifying factor they all have, is that all the processes involve boiling water to produce steam. This steam, in turn, takes along the healing properties and volatile qualities. After this, the condensation process occurs. This happens when the steam is chilled in a condenser. The result of this condensation is hydrosol- this is the distilled water with the oil floating on the surface. Afterward, the oil can be gotten from the hydrosol.

Steam Distillation

Steam distillation makes use of steam from an external source. This external steam is passed into the container where distillation takes place. This is done to hasten the extraction process and obtain as many compounds as possible. Once the external steam has gone into the section containing the plant content, it leaves the system through the condensing unit.

Hydrodistillation

In this process, the plant itself is soaked in hot water. This produces a sort of broth that has steam comprised of the healing molecules of the plant. This steam rising from the mixture is what is then condensed and used. This happens to be the oldest kind of distillation. One reason why it is so popular is that it leaves room for special kinds of modification. This method of distillation is still used in underdeveloped countries. It comes with its own risks, though. The still can dry up and end up burning the plant and invariably producing essential oil that has a burnt aroma.

Water and Steam Distillation

This process of distillation works like a sieving process. The contents of the plant and hot water are mixed. Then, this mixture is poured into a closed container that allows only steam to leave the container. This kind of distillation is very good for extracting compounds from leaves.

2. Solvent Extraction

There are some plant materials that are not strong enough to pass through the process of distillation- petals for instance. So, the best way to obtain their extracts is through solvent extraction. First, the section used for extraction is filled with the plant material. This section must be perforated. Then, the plant material is washed with a kind of solvent (solvents are liquids that dissolve solid, liquid and gaseous solutes, thus creating a solution). The solvent melts all the compounds from the plant that can be extracted. These compounds include non-aromatic, waxes, pigments and volatile molecules. After that, the solution gotten after washing the plant with the solvent is filtered. The undissolvable plant material is separated from the remaining solution. The filtrate, then, goes through a mild distillation to regain the solvent- this is done so that the solvent can be used for other solutions. What remains is a kind of wax. This is called concentrated concrete. This concrete goes through another type of processing to filter the authentic and unblemished essential oil from the wax. The process involves heating the wax and mixing it with alcohol. As this process is repeated, the concrete begins to change into a combination of liquid state and lumps. These lumps are separated from the liquid, which eventually becomes the finished product-essential oil.

3. Carbon Dioxide Extraction

When much pressure is applied to carbon dioxide, it moves from a gaseous state to a liquid form. In that case, carbon dioxide can be utilized as a solvent in absorbing the chemical compounds in the plant material through the process of solvent extraction. The upside is that there is never any form of lumps leftover from the solvent used in solvent extraction. So, once the carbon dioxide has done its job, it turns back to a gaseous state. Then, it dissipates into the air without any issues.

4. Cold Pressing/ Expression

Cold pressing is a form of extraction used for citrus fruits and plants. Naturally, the peels of citrus fruits are not strong enough to pass through distillation. They are also too loaded with healing compounds to be allowed to be washed by a solvent (regardless of the type). So, the oil is obtained through pressing. Much mechanical force is applied until the oil is obtained. This process is also known as expression.

5. Florasols/Phytols

This kind of oil extraction uses a different type of solvent in the extraction process. This process uses florasols as the solvent for drawing out the compounds of the plants. The first person to discover the capability of florasols in essential oil extraction was Dr. Peter Wilde. There is no application of heat in this extraction process as the whole activity takes place at room temperature. This kind of solvent leaves no room for residue or undissolvable plant materials. Every single part used in the process is utilized. There is no byproduct that emanates from this extraction process.

6. Enfleurage

This happens to be the most strenuous and costly way of obtaining essential oils. This is why it is seldom used. In the cases where the plants have very fragile parts that can be condemned by heat, enfleurage is the best way to get their essential oils. The plant materials are laid on sheets of warm fat. The fat then absorbs the oil in the plant. When all the oil has been gotten from the plant, it is removed from the sheets of fat and the next batch is placed on the fat. This is done until the fat is full of the essential oil it has extracted. Once this stage has been reached, alcohol is added to the fat to separate the fat from the oil. Then, the fat is used for other cosmetological products. The greatest upside of enfleurage is that it extracts every healing and chemical component that the plant is comprised of.

All these processes are the ways that oils can be extracted. Yet, with technological advances and new research on the essential oils, more processes are expected to come to the fore.

How Essential Oils Work

The key function of essential oils is to induce healing physically, mentally and emotionally. In fact, they have the capability to work like conventional pharmaceuticals. Sometimes, essential oils can heal at a faster and more effective date than normal drugs. How essential oils achieve this feat is what this chapter will be focused on.

Essential oils are comprised of certain chemical compounds that can heal any part of the body they are designed to heal. These compounds are encapsulated in molecules that have the ability to work their way into the body via the area where the body is exposed to the oils.

Experts have stated that essential oils are best used in two ways: inhaling and applying on the skin. Before using any essential oil at all, you should know that authentic essential oils are always very concentrated. This high level of concentration occurs because lots of plants are needed to obtain a small quantity of essential oil. So, whatever you do with the oils, make sure it is not superfluous.

The first means through which essential oils can work is what is known as inhalation (basically, smelling the oil). Inhalation can be done in three ways. You can just smell the oil by putting the bottle of essential oil close to your nose and just inhaling the scent directly. Inhalation can also be done by adding the diluted oil into a large bowl of hot water and tilting your head towards the oil-infused water (the process is called steaming). Then, you could get a diffuser that converts the oil into a gaseous form.

When the oil is inhaled, the molecules travel through the olfactory system and attach themselves to the smell receptors. This causes the nervous system to respond positively and begin the healing process. Experts have stated that this is the most efficient way to use essential oils. According to findings, the nerves in the olfactory system are directly linked to the brain. This ensures that the essential oil begins its work immediately the user inhales it.

The other means you can use an essential oil is by applying it to the skin. Experts call this "topical application". When you rub some essential oil on your skin, the molecules enter the body and circulatory system through the skin pores. The moment the healing compounds are in the bloodstream, they begin to make their way to the parts and organs of the body that they can heal. To make it easier and faster for the oils to start working, it is better to apply the oils to pulse points(areas where the arteries are close to the surface of the skin).

Also, massaging the point where the oil was placed will aid absorption. Some experts also claim that heat increases the rate of absorption of the essential oils into the body system. The end goal is for the oils to be absorbed into the body as soon as possible.

One final thing to note is that essential oils must always be diluted before they are used on the skin. As it was said earlier, essential oils in their pure form are usually very concentrated and potent. To this end, dermatologists and aromatherapists have advised that essential oils should be diluted with carrier oils such as sesame oil, olive oil, and canola oil. To fail to dilute essential oils before use is to flirt with danger.

To sum it all up, essential oils can be best used by inhaling or application on the skin. These methods of usage enable the molecules of the healing oils to move into the body and do their jobs.

Can Essential Oils Actually Cure Disease?

Essential oils have always been used and known for their healing properties. While there are many who claim that essential oils cannot cure diseases (just to keep Big Pharma happy), essential oils are capable of treating a significant number of diseases and health conditions. Many experts claim that there is not enough scientific evidence to prove that these oils work. They ignore the corpus of research on essential oils that was conducted in the 19th century spearheaded by René Maurice Gattefossé, Charles Chamberland and their contemporaries. They also ignore the recent research works on essential oils. They refuse to consider individuals that have asserted that essential oils worked for them. They refuse to conduct research on essential oils and they use the cases of people who failed to use the oils properly. To make matters worse, these cynics present these cases as the general results of using essential oils. Yet, all these things are of no consequence as essential oils are very much effective.

Subsequently, we will be exploring various essential oils and the kinds of health conditions they are used for.

Bergamot oil: This oil is gotten from the bergamot orange and its tree. The oil is extracted from the rinds, in particular. Bergamot oil has anti-inflammatory and anti-bacterial properties. Hence, it is very good for treating acne. It is also very good for treating pimples and black spots. When applying bergamot oil, you should dab the spot(s) that need treatment with the oil. Also, you should not go into the sun after using this essential oil. This oil also aids digestion. It frees up the respiratory system and it is very good for alleviating anxiety.

Chamomile oil: Chamomile oil is gotten from the chamomile plant (related to daisies). There are two kinds of chamomile plants. They are Roman chamomile and German chamomile. The core chemical compound in chamomile is chamazulene. German chamomile plants have a higher concentration of chamomile compared to Roman chamomile. Chamomile oil has been used since ancient times to cure colds and fevers. Chamomile oils are very good for dealing with nausea and they help out with insomnia. They are very effective pain relievers and they are often used to soothe the mind and calm the nerves.

Recent studies have shown that chamomile oil can be used to reduce depression, as well.

Clove oil: Clove oil is obtained from clove trees. The clove trees are usually found in the region of SouthEast Asia- you can find them in some other places, too. The clove oil is usually very light. It could be light yellow and it could be colorless- it depends on the time of extraction and the process, as well. Clove oil is very good for getting rid of bacteria. It helps with constipation and digestion problems. It also deals with respiratory issues such as asthma and cough. Clove oils are also very good for relieving toothaches.

Eucalyptus oil: Eucalyptus oil is gotten from the eucalyptus tree. The trees were primarily located in Australia. Now, they are grown all over the world. Eucalyptus oil is very useful for a number of things. Eucalyptus oil is very useful for stopping cough. Indeed, many cough syrups contain some portions of eucalyptus oil. It can also be used to remove mucus from the nostrils. In the end, this helps in curing catarrh. Eucalyptus oil also serves as an effective insect repellent. It can be used to disinfect wounds and it helps with bad breath (although you cannot put it in the mouth). Toothpaste and mouthwash producers always use eucalyptus oil to give their products that minty effect. It is also used as a great means to regulate blood sugar. Studies have also shown that eucalyptus oil can help with diabetes. In addition to this, eucalyptus oil helps with arthritis and joint pain.

Lavender oil: Lavender oil is one of the most effective and sought after essential oils. It is gotten from the lavender plant. Experts have stated that lavender oil has anti-inflammatory, antifungal, antidepressant, antiseptic, antibacterial and antimicrobial qualities. It can also be used as a sedative. Lavender oil also helps you feel relaxed. It is very useful for reducing menstrual pain. It reduces wrinkles and can sometimes be used as an anti-aging tool. It helps out with depression and it is very useful for treating wounds as it helps deal with inflammation. Lavender oil is also very good for insomnia and anxiety.

Lemon oil: Lemon oil is gotten from the fruit and parts of the lemon tree. It is widely known for its nice scent that lifts the spirits and energizes the body. Lemon oil has a wide range of uses. It is very good for detoxification. It clears the skin and rids of any unwanted things. It helps you focus and it is very useful for sharpening concentration skills. Lemon oil also elicits a positive mood from the user. It is an effective insect repellent. It makes the immune system stronger. Lemon oil has been known to help with weight loss and excess calories in the body system. Research has revealed that lemon oil helps with Alzheimer's disease, amongst other things.

Oregano oil: Oregano oil is gotten from the oregano plant. Oregano has many chemical compounds but the two most important compounds are carvacrol and thymol. These are the compounds that affect the work of oregano oil. It was the Greeks that first discovered this essential oil. They used it for treatment and day to day fashion activities. Oregano oil is very good for treating fungal infections. They help with irritation and bites. Oregano oil also strengthens the immune system. They help with fever and nausea. They are excellent for healing the skin. Oregano oils help with headaches, digestive problems.

Peppermint oil: Peppermint oil is a must-have for all users and lovers of essential oils. It is obtained from peppermint oil. It relaxes the muscles and relieves sore muscles. It cures colds and headaches. It is also very good for cramps, back pain, and menstrual pains.

Do essential oils cure diseases? This is a question whose answers many people do not want to hear. Essential oils cure diseases. They help in treating health conditions. They alleviate illnesses. Anyone looking to find something else apart from conventional medicine should try essential oils. They do work.

Chapter Five

Classification And Properties Of Some Essential Oils

There are hundreds of essential oils available and since it is quite difficult to know all of them, classifying them into families makes it easy to figure them out. When you're familiar with some of the basic families and the qualities that make them stand out, you'd not be overwhelmed when you are faced with a shelf of unknown oils.

Knowing the properties of these families should not prevent you from also learning about individual oils. The classification into families is meant to serve as a guide.

A. Floral and Floral Herbs

Some of the oils that are very common and familiar see grouped under this name. Florals include Jasmine, geranium, rose, neroli, ylang ylang, and many others. Many other flowering herbs like Clary sage, Roman chamomile, lavender can be called flowering oils because of their uses.

Florals are often very well rounded heady and sweet. If you can visualize a rose mid-bloom instead of the rosebud then you could understand that softness, but herbal floral is a little sharper. The floral family is made up of oils that can be used to balance hormones, stop depression or build romance. The floral oils are more suitable for hormonal issues like PMS, cramps and sleep disorders because of their balancing effect. Because of this strong effect, pregnant women are not meant to use them. The florals are also amazing when it comes to skincare because of the soothing effect.

Floral oils have a lot of benefits but they should not be used in all cases because they are heavy and can even constrict an already small room. If you need to remove smell from an environment, do not use floral oils because they often blend with scents instead of overpowering them or eliminating them.

Some of the floral oils include:

1. Rose

The scientific name is *Rosa damascena.*

Throughout history, it has been adored and admired both as an essential oil and a plant. The ancient Romans decorated their banquet halls and parties with a lot of roses. When Avicenna made the refrigerated coil part of the distillation process, the Rose plant was one of the first to be distilled.

Steam distillation or solvent extraction of rose flower petals will produce rose essential oil that has a spicy, rich, deep and sensual floral aroma. The scent is amazing but it uses goes beyond fragrance. For millenniums rose has been used in many natural beauty and health conditions.

Studies have shown that rose oil can reduce breathing rate, systolic blood pressure, and blood oxygen saturation. It helps relieve depression because of the flavonoids which contain antioxidants.

Rose oil is able to relieve oxidative stress and anxiety, fix certain skin problems, improve libido. It also contains natural compounds that improve general health and fights infection. Rose oil is made up of citronellol, nerol, and geraniol and it should not be used during pregnancy because it promotes the flow of blood in the pelvic area.

2. Lavender

The scientific name is *Lavandula angustifolia.*

For more than 2,500 years, lavender has been used in religion and medicine. Ancient Egyptians used it in making perfumes and mummies. The Romans cooked with it and perfumed the air. It was also used in their bath water which is why the plant got its name from the Latin "lavare" which means "to wash". Lavender oil is a common essential oil all over the world that is known for its versatility. It has relaxing properties that relieve tension and promote sleep. Lavender essential oil is gotten through steam distillation of lavender flowers. It has a calming and sweet floral aroma.

According to research lavender is able to reduce lab induced diabetes and maintain good body weight. Lavender is also used to provide relief for people with Alzheimer's. It lowers anxiety and depression and symptoms of post-traumatic stress disorder. Lavender also clears skin conditions and soothes burns and wounds. It reduces blood pressure and blood sugar.

It improves blood circulation, helps with respiratory disorders. People also use it to relieve sore muscles, headaches and boost libido. The active compounds in lavender are Alpha is Terpineol, Linalool, Linalyl acetate, and Beta Ocimene. The oil is easily tolerated by most people.

3. Geranium

The scientific name is *Pelargonium graveolens*.

Geranium has been used for a long time by the ancient Egyptians who used it to make their skin beautiful. The native Americans used geranium roots to make tea and drank it as natural medicine.

During the Victorian era, dining tables were covered with fresh geranium leaves and sometimes the edible parts of the plant were used as an ingredient for cakes, dessert, and jellies.

In this era, geranium is included in various treatment methods. It helps to improve mental, emotional and physical health with its antidepressant, healing and antiseptic properties. Geranium essential oils are extracted by steam distillation from the stalks and leaves of the plant.

According to research, geranium is able to suppress Candida cell growth and hemorrhage episodes.

Geranium can be used for various skin conditions, to stabilize hormones, reduce depression and mood swings. It is an antifungal oil that reduces blood pressure and helps with symptoms of menopause. It heals inflammation and stress, maintains oil production and also serves as an anti-stress agent. The active compounds in geranium are citronellol and geraniol. Women in their first trimesters are not advised to use the oil. They may use it later on in topical dilutions. Also, people with sensitive skin should be careful with it.

B. Citrus Oils

The citruses are a well known essential oil family. It includes commonly known orange, bergamot and lemon and less commonly known, lime, grapefruit, and mandarin.

Almost everyone can recognize a citrus scent and it is often used in cleaning. Citrus oils are sweet and fresh but they do not have the same heavy sweetness of some florals and vanilla.

Citrus oils are your best bet when you're feeling low and gloomy. They help with mood disorders and lethargy. It has detoxification and energy-boosting properties. They are a wonderful choice for removing bad smells and they easily appeal to most people.

Citrus oils are often phototoxic and so they may cause reactions when you use them on your body and go into the sun. Use pre-made blends if you want to prevent that effect.

Some of the citrus oils are:

1. Bergamot

The scientific name is *Citrus bergamia*.

This oil originates in southeast Asia. The evergreen citrus tree is cold-pressed and distilled to produce the oil. Some Bergamot trees can be found in Algeria, Morocco, Ivory Coast, and Tunisia.

The taste is somewhat like a hybrid between a lemon and sour orange.

Bergamot is a unique citrus oil because it is able to uplift and calm the soul. It helps the skin with purification and cleansing. Bergamot is an antibacterial agent that can relieve headaches, heal scars and muscle pain. It also helps to improve the hormonal and digestive juices and keep them flowing.

According to research, bergamot oil treats anxiety and depression. It is known for reducing blood pressure and pulse rate and soothe body tension. Apart from being antibacterial, bergamot is antiseptic and antifungal. It is a natural deodorant that also helps balance oily skin. When using bergamot, stay away from direct sunlight for about 12 hours after topical use. It may also affect your blood sugar levels so diabetics should use it with caution. The active compounds in bergamot are Limonene, Linalyl formate, and Linalool.

2. Orange

The scientific name is *Citrus sinensis*.

There is a fascinating and mythical history surrounding Orange. The Japanese connected citrus blossoms to a state of chastity. The Arab women used it as a dye for their grey hair. Nostradamus made writings on how to make cosmetics from its fruit and blossoms. It was so valuable to Hercules that he stole it from Hesperides who kept it as the main food for ancient Roman and Greek gods.

One interesting fact about sweet orange is that it is not a wild plant and it is believed to be a hybrid product of the mandarin (Citrus reticulata) and the pummelo (Citrus maxima). The essential oil from orange is gotten from cold pressing the outer peel of the fruit.

Orange essential oil is beneficial for its antidepressant, anti-cancer, antibacterial properties.

The citrusy aroma of orange oil boosts the emotions and eliminates stress.

According to research, the flavonoid antioxidants in orange could stop the growth of some cancer cells.

Orange benefits include detoxification, reduction of anxiety, and reduction of wrinkles. People also use orange oil for treating cold and flu symptoms, improving circulation and blood pressure. It also helps with lymphatic drainage and boosting energy. The active compound in the orange essential oil is Limonene, Myrcene. There should be no direct exposure to sunlight for 12 hours after applying the oil. Since orange oil may cause sensitive reactions, it is best to test it on a small portion of the skin.

3. Lemon

The scientific name is *Citrus limon.*

The lemon essential oil has been used in Ayurvedic medicine for a long time to treat several health conditions. The traditional Chinese health practitioners use lemon peel oil for its ability to fight conditions like loose stools, Candida, common cold, sore throat, and other respiratory conditions. It also improves liver health and provides natural relief for gallstones. The active compound also has anti-cancer properties. Lemon oil detoxifies the body and stimulates lymph drainage, boosts energy and clears the skin.

Lemon essential oil is extracted from the rind of the lemon by cold pressing. The extracted oil has a sweet, citrusy scent that uplifts and refreshes.

Some studies have shown that lemon oil reduces pregnancy-related nausea and fights stress.

Lemon oil is used to freshen the breath, suppress cough, aid the body in fat digestion and lymphatic drainage. It is also an antidepressant, antifungal, antibacterial, antiseptic and anti-anxiety agent. Lemon oil aids in weight loss, digestion and can induce deep sleep during the daytime.

C. Trees

This family is made up of oils derived from trees although not every oil extracted from a tree is included. The members of this family - tea tree, cedarwood, eucalyptus and all evergreen trees like cypress, pine, and fir all have some shared qualities. To familiarize yourself with the qualities of this family, think of eucalyptus as the poster child.

Oils in this family are good for cases of flu, colds allergies, and other respiratory issues. Upon inhalation of any of the oils in this family, the nose and chest experience a cooling sensation and that's what makes them right for congestion, sinus irritation, allergies, and coughs.

Not only that, but tree oils are also antibacterial and some of them prevent infection of wounds. This makes them the perfect choice for clearing acne.

These oils produce a cooling effect in the circulatory system and are often used in pain reduction blend. Oils from this family can induce muscle relaxation and release body tension. Other benefits of these oils include panic attacks and anxiety relief. Oils in this family mask and eliminate bad odors in the environment. They provide energy and also encourage good sleep. Some members of this family are:

1. Eucalyptus

The scientific name is *Eucalyptus radiata*.

There is a story in English folklore about an early English settler who almost severed his thumb with an ax. His father who had knowledge of aboriginal folk medicine suggested a bandage made from eucalyptus leaves. When he showed the wound to a surgeon later, he was surprised that the thumb healed fast without being infected.

The tree is also called Tasmanian Blue Gum and it is native to Australia. People see eucalyptus as the main food for Koala bears. Despite being a source of nutrition for wildlife, eucalyptus essential oil with its cool, crisp fragrance has strong therapeutic uses. Eucalyptus oil is extracted by steam distillation of the leaves and twigs.

According to some studies, eucalyptus oil can reduce pain, inflammation, and swelling. Eucalyptus oil improves breathing by opening the airways and it makes massage even more soothing. The oil serves as a disinfectant, energizer, and deodorant. The oil fights infection and enhances mental clarity. It boosts the respiratory system, provides energy and is an antibacterial, antiseptic and anti-anxiety agent. Eucalyptus oil is also used to combat fever, earaches and some skin problems. The active compound in eucalyptus oil is Alpha Terpineol and Eucalyptol.

2. Tea Tree

The scientific name is *Melaleuca alternifolia*. Some people call it Melaleuca. Knowledge of these oils has been handed down for millenniums by the Bundjalung aborigines of Australia. The people used spiritual medicine mainly for major illnesses but the tea tree plant was used for common issues. According to the legend, tea tree leaves had been falling into a certain "mystical" lake for centuries so much that the mud was made up of concentrated tea tree oil. They applied the mud on their skin as medicine.

Melaleuca is well recognized for being an antiseptic and being able to heal injuries.

Several medical research has been carried out on melaleuca for more than 70 years because of its ability to destroy some strains of viruses, bacteria, and fungi. Tea tree oil is extracted from the steam distillation of the melaleuca plant. The oil has a fresh earthy, medicinal and woody scent that purifies and cleanses.

Studies have shown that tea tree oil was able to treat acne in a number of patients and it also provided a remedy for yeast infections in cancer patients.

Tea tree oil is an antibacterial, anti-fungal, antiviral and antiseptic natural deodorant. It destroys lice, boosts the circulatory and respiratory system, and provides relief for earaches. It is also a good treatment for cold sores and skin blemishes. It energizes the body and relieves anxiety and is also good at balancing oily skin. It can also be used in oral health to prevent bad breath but should never be congested or used internally for any reason. When used as a mouth wash or toothpaste, the oil should be spat out to avoid harmful side effects like hives, digestive issues or dizziness. The active component includes Alpha- & Y-Terpinenes, Terpinen-4-ol, and P-Cymene.

3. Cedarwood

The scientific name is Cedrus atlantica.

Throughout history, cedarwood has been used for medicinal purposes. The ancient Egyptians used both the wood and oil for embalmment. The tree is quite related to the Cedar of Lebanon repeatedly mentioned in the Bible. There is a large grove of Lebanese cedars on the slopes of Mount Lebanon. The oil gives off a relaxing, woody aroma. Cedarwood essential oil is extracted from the wood of the cedarwood tree by steam distillation.

Cedarwood is able to improve the functioning of organs, enhance the digestive system and metabolism, soothe the skin and muscles. This is probably why the Bible made mention of cedars more than other trees because they symbolized wisdom, protection, and abundance.

Studies have shown that cedarwood essential oil could help boost the learning abilities of children with ADHD.

Cedarwood oil is an antibacterial, antifungal and antiseptic substance. It promotes healthy skin by relieving some skin conditions like psoriasis and eczema. It enhances the respiratory and circulatory systems. It helps with sleep and anxiety disorders, relaxes the muscles, improves menstruation, fights cough and is also a deodorant.

The active compounds in cedarwood oil are Beta-cedrene, Alpha-cedrene, Cedrol. This oil is not safe for internal use and during pregnancy. It is advisable to dilute before topical use.

D. Herbs

This family is not comprised of all herbs. The herbs that are part of this group are known for their delicious scent that is somewhat similar to oils from the tree family. Some of the herbs in this family include basil, peppermint, rosemary, sage, spearmint, etc.

There are only very few similarities between the members of this family.

Herbal oils are also antibacterial and antifungal that help with respiratory issues.

These oils are able to improve blood circulation, they have detoxification abilities, helps to relieve tension and relax muscles, and they help in digestion. Using herbal oils can increase your energy, help improve concentration and memory. They also act as deodorants. They include:

1. Peppermint

The scientific name is *Mentha piperita*. It is among the oldest European medicinal herbs. It uses dates back to the medicinal practices of ancient Chinese, Japanese and Egyptians. Ancient Greeks used it in funerals. In Biblical times, it was mentioned along with cumin and anise to be used as a tithe offering to the lord.

Peppermint was discovered in the 17th century and said to be a cross between some types of wild mints. Peppermint essential oil is extracted from the steam distillation of the whole plant. The essential oil has anti-nausea benefits. it soothes the muscles, gastric lining, and colon. The sharp minty scent provides a cooling sensation on the body that relieves headaches and sore muscles on topical use. It is also an antimicrobial and so can aid digestion. It is an anti-inflammatory, anti-fungal, antibacterial, antidepressant, anti-anxiety, energizer and pain relief. The active compounds in peppermint are menthone and menthol.

2. Basil

The scientific name is *Ocimum basilicum.*

It is an ancient herb that is found mostly in Egyptian pyramids. In the past, ancient kings were anointed with basil on special occasions. Asians used basil to produce venom for some insects and snakes. Basil is a sacred plant in India because it is planted in graves and temples. Chinese and Ayurvedic medicine practitioners treated flu, colds fever earaches and muscle aches with basil. Some hundreds of years ago, basil scent was known to be alluring and Italian women wore the oil and put it around them just to lure suitors.

Basil essential oil is often referred to as "sweet basil oil". It is gotten from the steam distillation of the Ocimum basilicum plant. The sweet, spicy warm and herbal scent of basil is not only favored for its use as a flavor enhancer. It is also used to heal various infections and wounds. It is an anti-inflammatory agent that also alleviates muscle and nerve conditions.

Basil was regarded as a sacred plant by certain religious texts like that of the Hindu.

According to Ayurveda, basil helps to increase spiritual awareness. The plant is called an adaptogen because it can stimulate or sedate depending on which one the body needs.

The essential oil is gotten through steam distillation of the leaves and flowers.

Some studies showed that basil was able to inhibit the growth of *Staphylococcus aureus* and *Escherichia coli*.

Basil is antibacterial, anti-inflammatory, antioxidant and anti-anxiety. It helps with adrenal fatigue and lung disorders. It improves respiratory health and helps to regulate blood sugar levels. It stimulates the nervous system and helps reduce ear infections and acne. It helps with memory retention and digestion and provides relief for muscle spasm.

People with impaired liver function should be careful while using oils with the main compound of basil, eugenol. Also, eugenol should be avoided in patients with clotting disorders because of its anticoagulant properties. Basil should not be used during pregnancy or in epileptic patients.

3. Rosemary

The scientific name is *Rosmarinus officinalis*.

For a long time, Rosemary has been used to boost natural health. Rosemary tea was used to soothe the nerves, improve memory and make perfumes.

Right from 1584, Rosemary was used for remembrance of occasions like weddings or funeral.

In Hamlet, Shakespeare made mention of Rosemary where Ophelia was serenaded by flowers and says "Rosemary is for remembrance. Even in earlier years, it was still regarded as a sacred herb by the ancient Romans, Greeks, and Egyptians.

Rosemary was used all over to cleanse the air and prevent the spread of illness in the air. In ancient medicine, it was used to improve memory, soothe muscle ailments and tackle digestive problems. Recently, Rosemary has been used to effectively boost nerves and brain function. The essential oil is extracted from steam distillation of the plant leaves and it exudes a woody, fresh scent.

According to studies, Rosemary affects the mood and cognitive performance of individuals. They have been found to be antibacterial especially against most pathogenic bacteria including drug-resistant *E. coli*. It is also an anti-fungal. It is an anti-inflammatory that helps in reducing pain and settling most respiratory concerns. It can be used to improve hair growth. Rosemary works as an antidepressant and a hormone booster.

Rosemary oil should be used with caution in pregnant women or people with high blood pressure, and epilepsy. The active compounds are 1,8-cineole, Linalool, Terpinen-4-ol.

E. Resins

Resins are very easy to recognize with the exception of a few. They are often deep base notes and while some have a musky scent others have a sweet scent. Members of this group include oakmoss, patchouli, sandalwood, myrrh, vetiver, and benzoin.

When they are put in bottles, the oils look dark and thick and It is quite hard to get them out. Resins are often extracted by the resinoid solvent method with the exception of a few.

Resins are among the oils recommended mostly for anxiety, stress and panic attacks. They provide a grounding effect and keep your body together. They help with deep relaxation, slow heartbeats, and calm racing thoughts. They even act as antidepressants especially frankincense which people know as the best oils for that disorder.

People use most of the resins as aphrodisiacs especially sandalwood and patchouli. Resins are also known for soothing skin disorders like irritations, dryness, and itching from psoriasis and eczema. Many of them are antibacterial, anti-inflammatory, antifungal and suitable for respiratory issues.

Some of them are:

1. Patchouli

The scientific name is *Pogostemon cablin.*

Patchouli was famous as a moth repellent in the 19th century when the Indians used it in clothing that they exported. Before long, the scent was used to indicate a true fabric from the "orient" that even the English and French clothmakers became jealous and used the patchouli scent on their imitation products so that people would accept their goods in the domestic market.

People practicing traditional medicine in China, Malaysia, and Japan have used patchouli oil for some remedies. It has been known to be a cell rejuvenator used for healing wounds and scars. People also used it to treat insect and snake bites. Patchouli essential oil is produced by steam distillation of the leaves.

Patchouli leaves are put through a steam distillation process to extract the essential oil. The strong scent of patchouli oil has been used for centuries in perfumes; more recently it's been used in incense, insect repellents, and natural remedies. Patchouli is considered a great balancer, relaxing yet stimulating, particularly relevant for conditions of weak immunity. Patchouli is known to treat various skin conditions, such as acne and inflammation. It also has anti-fungal, digestive and antiseptic properties. According to a study, the anti-inflammatory activity is able to prevent cancer initiation. Patchouli is a deodorant, hair growth booster, antidepressant, aphrodisiac, and immune booster. The active compounds in patchouli are AlphaPinene and Sabinene. If you are on any prescribed drugs, it will be best to discuss with your healthcare practitioner before using it because it may inhibit blood clotting.

2. Sandalwood

The scientific name is Santalum album.

Sandalwood has a unique intoxicating and Woody scent.

The Hindus have for many thousands of years employed sandalwood in their important religious ceremonies. The Egyptians used it for medicinal purposes, for embalmment of their dead, and veneration of their gods.

Sandalwood is originally from the Asian tropics, is an evergreen tree and can even grow to reach 30 feet. The more mature a sandalwood tree is, the more fragrance and quality it has. The essential oil is very therapeutic, can improve clarity and make the body calmer. The sandalwood essential oil is extracted through steam distillation of the wood. The oil improves meditation and balances the cardiovascular system.

Studies have shown that sandalwood can be anticancerous without having toxic effects.

Sandalwood is a natural aphrodisiac, an antidepressant, and anti-anxiety. It soothes the muscle, removes cramps and breaks us mucus and congestion. Use sandalwood only after dilution with a carrier oil.

3. Frankincense

The scientific name can be Boswellia Frereana, Boswellia Carterii, Boswellia Sacra depending on the species.

Frankincense is referred to as the king of oils and is very potent, therapeutic and effective.

For centuries people have used frankincense in their religious practices, meditation, and worship. Frankincense is a small shrub or tree that has a lot of pinnate leaves with white or pinkish flowers.

Frankincense produces a natural oleo gum resin that can be drained out by creating cuts in the back. The resin then undergoes steam distillation to produce the essential oil.

Frankincense is a very precious essential oil with amazing health values. It reduces, anxiety, pain, and inflammation and can be a suitable remedy for chronic stress. It helps to fight against tumors and strengthen the body's immunity.

Frankincense possesses sesquiterpenes that allow it to travel beyond the blood-brain barrier. It is also able to intensify the activities of leukocytes and increase the body's ability to fight infections. According to a study, frankincense oil is able to cause the death of breast cancer cells and it can also work as an anti-inflammatory.

This oil is able to rejuvenate skin and prevent aging, improve the hormone levels of the body, support immunity, and aid respiration. Frankincense is an anti-anxiety, antidepressant, antiseptic, and sedative. It helps digestion, calms the body and increases focus. The active compounds in frankincense are AlphaPinene, Limonene, and AlphaThujene.

Frankincense should be used with care because it has blood-thinning effects. Patients with blood clotting issues should see their health care practitioner before using the oil.

F. Spices

Only very few spice oils are familiar and common. The more popular ones are cinnamon, ginger, and clove, cassia bark, and nutmeg.

It is very easy to recognize spice oils because of their spicy scent. They produce a hot feeling when ingested and can either smell like medicine or fresh baking depending on the quantity in any blend.

Essential oils in this family are often very beneficial for cases of flu and cold. They are more often used for their antifungal, antibacterial, and efficiency with respiratory issues. This family is the best choice for relieving digestive issues.

Spice oils are hot and when they are used in massage oils they can reduce inflammation, stimulate circulation and bring relief to pain. Oils in this family should be used carefully because they can cause painful rash or burns when they are used without being diluted or they are at a low dilution. Using spice oils in small quantities can give you a feeling of comfort and safety. however, making blends with high percentages of spice oils can be too stimulating and cause irritation to the lungs and nasal passages. Some examples of spice oils include:

1. Cinnamon

The scientific name is *Cinnamomum verum.*

Cinnamon has been used by Egyptians in their embalmment process for a very long time. The Holy Bible even mentioned cinnamon as an ingredient of the holy anointing oil.

According to legend, emperor Nero burned at much cinnamon as he could lay his hands on the pyre which he used to bury his second wife Poppaea Sabina in A.D. 65 as atonement for the part he played in her death.

The outer bark of the cinnamon tree is processed through steam distillation to obtain cinnamon bark oil.

For thousands of years, people have used cinnamon oil for the medicinal properties it possesses. Cinnamon bark has a warm and strong scent that can stimulate the senses.

Cinnamon oil contains antioxidants that can help to improve the digestive system, stabilize blood sugar and help blood circulation. It is often used as a remedy for cardiovascular disease and for combating infections.

Cinnamon oil is an anti-inflammatory, anti-fungal and anti-bacterial. It may be useful in curbing depression and fighting some antiviral diseases. It is sometimes used as an aphrodisiac and pain reducer.

The active compounds in cinnamon oil are Eugenol, Cinnamaldehyde 117, Phellandrene, and Methyleugenol.

2. Clove

The scientific name is *Eugenia caryophyllata*.

The Chinese have used clove for more than 2000 years as a spice and fragrance and even now, its usage has spread across the world. It has been used in making several products for controlling pests and making cosmetics.

Clove was used as a love potion by the Persians during ancient times. Research has shown us that clove has high antioxidant properties that make our lives better.

They appear in nature as the closed pink flower buds of the evergreen clove tree. After steam distillation of the buds, the essential oil is extracted and it produces a warm spicy scent.

Clove oil has been used in traditional medicine because of its versatility. It contains high levels of eugenol and has been used as an effective alternative or supplement to some modern remedies.

Clove oil has been researched to have bactericidal and fungicidal properties. Using this oil will help to promote healthy gums, protect the skin and mucous membranes and boost energy. It improves respiration and stops congestion. It reduces the symptoms of osteoporosis and is anti-anemic. The active compound in clove is eugenol. It is advisable to dilute clove oil before topical use. For internal use, clove oil should not be used for more than two consecutive weeks. It's also necessary to include probiotic supplement twice daily to replenish the important flora.

3. Ginger

The scientific name is *Zingiber officinale*.

Ginger was an expensive commodity way back in the 14th century. It cost almost the same as a live sheep but thankfully now, due to its widespread use in herbal medicine almost everyone can afford it. Ginger is present in the delicacies of most Asians with its hot, fragrant aroma. The westerners use it to make sweets and snacks like gingerbread and ginger snaps. The ginger oil is extracted through steam distillation of the roots and it gives off a warm and pleasant aroma.

Ginger is easily the most used herb in Chinese medicine because it's warming properties makes it the best choice for lowering the body's internal dampness.

Ginger is more potent when it is an essential oil because that's when the gingerol levels are at its highest. Gingerol is a strong anti-inflammatory, antiseptic, anti-nausea and warming agent. It relieves menstrual disorder, reduces pain and helps boost the respiratory and circulatory system.

It also gives the user a sense of courage and self-assurance. The active compounds in ginger are Gingerol and AlphaZingiberene. People with sensitive skin are advised to dilute the oil before using it.

Other essential oils

1. Birch

The scientific name is *Betula lenta*

Birch essential oil is also called sweet birch oil. It contains methyl salicylate and has been known as a suitable treatment for sore and tired muscles.

The chemical composition of birch oil is similar to those of wintergreen essential oil and that's the reason why the American Indians and the first European settlers made their tea with both birch bark and wintergreen because they wanted to get their stimulating and warming properties.

The native Americans used birch to solve health problems like dysentery, indigestion, and diarrhea.

The scent produced by birch oil is minty and earthy and it is used to heal muscle pain and boost awareness.

Birch essential oil is extracted from the steam distillation of the birch tree. Its chemical components make it the best choice for improving skin health.

According to research, birch oil possesses antibacterial properties and can provide potent treatment for precancerous skin conditions.

It provides support for the respiratory system and relieves tendonitis and arthritis. It can also relieve cramps and balance emotions. The active compounds in birch oil are Betulene, Methylsalicyclate, and butilinol. Birch oil is not recommended for use by pregnant or nursing mothers, people with ADD/ADHD, seizure disorder, salicylate deficiency, bleeding disorders or those taking blood thinners. It should be diluted before topical use.

2. Black Pepper

The scientific name is *Piper nigrum.*

From archaeological reports, pepper has been used in India since 2000 B.C.

There are Greek and Roman texts that indicate there was pepper trade between India and the West. The Romans loved to cook with pepper, so much that 80 percent of their recipes contained pepper as a spice.

It has also been discovered that India and Egypt traded pepper. When Ramsey the great of Egypt was mummified, peppercorns were stuffed into his nose.

The fruits of the black pepper are processes through steam distillation to extract the pepper essential oil.

The oil has a peppery, warm and spicy scent. It is often used for issues relating to the digestive and nervous systems. It promotes circulation and improves emotion. Black pepper not only opens the senses, but it also boosts mental clarity.

According to some studies, black pepper oil can fight some smoking withdrawal symptoms and reduce pain.

Black pepper helps to improve the flavor of food and digestion. It increases energy and provides relief for spasms and cramps. It is anti-anxiety, anti-inflammatory and antispasmodic. The active compound in black pepper is Carene, Limonene, and Caryophyllene.

Dilute the oil before using it topically.

3. Cardamom

The scientific name is *Elettaria cardamomum.*

This essential oil was among the spices adored by the ancient Greeks and Romans.

The Egyptians also used it in making medicines, for embalmment and other rituals.

They cleaned their teeth and freshened their breath by chewing the pods. Cardamom has been used as a medicine for colds, diarrhea, gas and kidney problems, colic, nausea, and reproductive troubles.

The essential oil is extracted by steam distillation of seeds that have been dried for more than three months. It's versatility and the spicy, sweet and balsamic scent which it exudes makes it a favorite spice for most people around the world.

The scent is soothing and helps to improve mental function, focus and reduce drowsiness. According to research, cardamom oil has some anti-inflammatory and antibacterial properties. It aids digestion and helps the body to relax. It might be useful in alleviating menopausal symptoms, cramps, and spasms.

The active compounds in cardamom are Linalool, 1,8-cineole, and terpinyl acetate. People with sensitive skin can get allergic reactions from using cardamom. Avoid using cardamom on the face of infants or young children.

4. Cassia

The scientific name is *Cinnamomum cassia.*

Traditional Chinese medicine regards cassia as one of its 50 fundamental herbs. The Chinese sold cassia to the Egyptians for them to use in their embalming process.

People in the ancient Middle East adored cassia so much that it was equivalent to gold or ivory.

The Bible mentions Cassia severally as anointing oil.

The cassia's plant's bark, twigs, and leaves are processed through steam distillation to produce cassia essential oil.

The scent is spicy and warm, almost like cinnamon but sweeter.

In traditional medicine, cassia oil is used to treat leprosy, cough, tuberculosis, ulcer symptoms, menstrual problems, erysipelas, and flatulence. It is also used commonly as a supportive treatment for anemia, constipation, and bronchitis.

According to research, cassia oil is able to prevent plaques from forming in the arteries. Also, it has been seen to have antibacterial and antifungal effects.

Cassia functions as an astringent, improves blood circulation and boosts the immune system. It is used to stabilize blood sugar, provide relief for menstrual symptoms and help people with depression. The active compounds in cassia oil are Cinnamyl acetate and Cinnamaldehyde. When taken internally, cassia should be used only in small doses. It could lower milk production in lactating women.

5. Cilantro

The scientific name is *Coriandrum sativum.*

Cilantro has been used for both culinary uses and other benefits for several years. Cilantro seeds have been discovered in caves that were used in ancient Israel.

For centuries, cilantro has been used in Europe, North Africa, the Middle East, and Asia, for that fresh tang and its medicinal properties. It has been known to help fight some fungi and bacteria.

In today's world, Americans use cilantro and cilantro oils to prepare liver detoxification supplements because they are able to clean the liver and carry out general body detoxification by removing heavy metals like lead and mercury.

The oil is extracted through steam distillation of the leaves. The oil has a slight citrus scent and fresh flavor. Cilantro oil is very similar to coriander oil because while cilantro is distilled from the leaf of Coriandrum sativum, coriander oil is extracted from the seed of the same plant. Upon topical application, cilantro cools and soothes the skin. When used to make an essential oil blend, it adds that fresh, herbal aroma to it.

From research, Coriandrum sativum has been able to improve the function of the liver and help treat diabetes. It also works as a detoxifier and cleanses the body of heavy metal deposits.

It eases gas, bloating and indigestion. Cilantro oil is anti-inflammatory, anti-fungal and anti-bacterial. It also helps to fight allergies and clear the mind.

The active compound in cilantro oil is Decenal and dodecenal. Generally, cilantro oil is not toxic or irritating, or sensitive.

6. Citronella

The scientific name is *Cymbopogon nardus.*

Hearing the word citronella often reminds us of how our citronella candles help to chase bugs away. Citronella is famous for being a good insect repellent but that's not all it is good for.

Chinese medical practitioners used citronella to bring relief for muscle aches and joint pain. Also, citronella has a really strong calming effect. It scents a little like citrus and possesses antiseptic, antibacterial and anti-fungal properties. Citronella oil is extracted by steam distillation of the plant's stems and leaves. It contains phytochemicals and antioxidants and has been widely used in Sri Lanka, Indonesia, and China for centuries to stop inflammation, reduce rashes and infections and treat other conditions.

Citronella is beneficial to the respiratory system and helps to achieve a relaxed state. It repels insects and removes free radicals. It is an anti-inflammatory, antiseptic, antibacterial, antifungal and is able to heal muscle pain.

Citronella should be diluted before use because it may be sensitive to the skin. The active compounds are citronellal, geraniol, and citronellol.

7. Clary Sage

The scientific name is *Salvia sclarea.*

Medieval author's referred to the herb as "clear eye". They thought it useful for eye-related issues. "clary" is gotten from the Latin word for clear, "Clarus".

People of the middle ages referred to it as "Oculus Christi," or the "eyes of Christ."

Sage is known in Chinese medicine as a herb that boosts the kidneys, female reproductive organs, and adrenals.

It is among the herbs that are recommended mostly for balancing women's hormones.

It helps to treat cramps, hormonal imbalance, heavy menstrual cycle, and hot flashes. Clary Sage essential oil is gotten from steam distillation of the flower and the scent is quite musky but feminine.

Clary Sage oil is one of the most soothing, relaxing and grounding essential oils. It can provide comfort and good sleep for those who inhale it. It is also able to support the circulatory system, digestive system, and the eye.

According to research, Clary Sage oil is able to reduce the feeling of pain, anxiety and the fear accompanied by labor. Also, it was found to have antimicrobial properties and prevent skin and wound infections.

Clary Sage improves mood, reduces stress, and helps to relieve asthma symptoms. Apart from being antibacterial, it is also anti-fungal and antiseptic.

The active compounds in Clary sage oil are linalool, Germacrene-D, Linalyl acetate. The sage oil is advisable for use by pregnant women in their first trimester because it can induce uterine contractions.

8. Coriander

The scientific name is *Coriandrum Sativum.*

Coriander has been used for a long time in the past. Based on historical findings, coriander seeds were located in the ancient tomb of Egyptian Ramses the Great. The plant can also be used as a spice especially the leaves and seeds.

Coriander essential oil is extracted through steam distillation of the seeds of the Coriandrum plant. The other parts of the plant are used to make cilantro essential oil.

This oil has a sweet, woody and spicy scent. For several centuries, coriander has been used to improve the hormonal and digestive systems. It is also able to provide a calming effect and ease us of the stress accompanied with our daily hectic life.

According to a study, coriander is able to combat fungal infections and pathogenic bacteria.

It provides relief for stomach problems, migraine headaches. It is a sedative and helps to reduce muscle and joint pain. It supports blood circulation and helps to maintain a healthy insulin response.

The active compounds in coriander essential oil are Linalool and Terpenes. People with sensitive skin should dilute coriander before using topically.

9. Cumin

The scientific name is *Cuminum Cyminum.*

In the past Egyptians used cumin to prepare foods and also preserve their mummies. The Romans and Greeks used cumin to spice their foods and make medicine.

Also, they used it to turn their complexion pale. The traditional Middle Easterns use cumin as a spice. It is a major component of curry and also used to form hummus.

People in France use cumin oil to treat some chronic viral diseases because of the antiviral properties of its aldehyde, cuminal.

The oil is gotten from the steam distillation of dried and crushed cumin seeds. Cumin oil boosts the immune and nervous systems. It helps the cardiovascular system to function properly. The earthy and spicy scent of cumin can improve The digestive system and boost appetite by stimulating bowel movement. It has antiparasitic, antiviral, antibacterial, and antioxidant properties.

Cumin oil is able to regulate menstruation and detoxify the body. It releases stress and anxiety, tones the muscles, skin, and tissues and is able to prevent gas.

The active compounds in cumin essential oil are Cuminic acids, Cymene, BetaPinene Alpha- and Y-Terpinenes. Cumin oil should not be used during pregnancy because it can spike blood flow to the uterus. After applying cumin oil externally, stay away from direct sunlight.

10. Cypress

The scientific name is *Cupressus sempervirens.*

Cypress was used by the early Cretans and Phoenicians to build houses and ships. The Egyptians made sarcophagi from it to bury their dead while the Greeks used it to carve statues of the gods they worshipped.

Cypress got its name from the Greek word for "ever-living". Many art and literature work cited cypress trees to be an emblem of death, some legends even say that the cross on which Jesus was crucified was made from cypress.

Even though it symbolizes sorrowful things, cypress is famous for its fragrance and the relaxing oil extracted from it. The oil is cherished for its ability in fighting infections, detoxifying the body, boosting the respiratory system and relieving anxiety.

The essential oil is extracted from the steam distillation of young twigs, needles, and stems from the cypress tree. The oil produced from cypress has a clean, woody and energizing scent. It also contains monoterpenes which makes it a good choice for clearing oily skin conditions.

According to studies cypress oil can be antibacterial and anti-fungal.

It is a mood booster and relieves muscle pain. It has deodorant, antiseptic and antibacterial properties. It provides relief for carpal tunnel syndrome and may reduce cellulite and varicose veins. The active compounds in cypress oil are Carene, Limonene, and AlphaPinene. Cypress oil should not be used during pregnancy.

11. Fennel

The botanical name is *Foeniculum vulgare*.

Fennel has been used since ancient times by Roman warriors who consumed it as a way of getting stronger and preparing for battle.

Many cultures have harnessed the medicinal properties of fennel.

In Chinese traditional medicine, fennel was used to treat lots of health problems—from soothing congestion to boosting the production of breast milk.

Fennel is a winter vegetable that looks like celery and has an exotic flavor and scent.

The oil is extracted from steam distillation of crushed fennel seeds and the scent can provide a supportive and purifying feeling.

Fennel can be used to soothe exhausted muscles and joints after workouts or a busy day.

Fennel has antitoxic, antiseptic and antioxidant properties. It can help to relieve digestive conditions, menstrual conditions, and PMS. It reduces nausea, colic, cramps, and spasms. The active compounds in fennel are Benzene, Anethole, and Limonene. Fennel should not be used by pregnant women and people who are either epileptic or prone to seizures. Also, it should not be used internally for a long time. Fennel should be diluted before using topically to avoid skin irritation.

12. Fir Needle

The scientific name is *Abies balsamea.*

Fir needle teases our imaginations to produce scenes of an exotic winter fantasy land. However, fir trees and oil provide both enjoyment and good health.

In some cultures, the fir tree is known as "forest healer" because of its healing properties.

Native Americans made paddling pillows from fir needles to allow them to sleep peacefully. It was also used to prevent disease in women after childbirth. The fir needles are the velvety, flat, needle-like leaves of the tree and they pass through steam distillation to produce fir needle essential oil. The important and active compounds in a fir tree are found in the needle.

The aroma of the oil extracted from the tree is fresh, earthy and woody. It is mostly used to combat respiratory diseases and sore throat, muscle aches, fatigue, and arthritis.

According to studies, fir needle has some anti-tumor characteristic that makes it a potential natural cancer treatment. Also, it was discovered to be antioxidant and antibacterial.

Fir needle is beneficial because it helps to stop symptoms of rheumatism, and arthritis pain. It can be a treatment for sinusitis and cold and flu symptoms. It improves bone health and helps with muscle aches. The active compounds in fir needle are AlphaPinene, Limonene, Camphene, and Tricyclene. Dilute fir needle oil before topical application to prevent skin sensitivity.

13. Grapefruit

The scientific name is *Citrus X Paradise.*

People refer to it as one of the seven wonders of Barbados and the forbidden fruit.

The first documentation of grapefruit was in 1750 by Welshman Rev. Griffith Hughes. It got its name "grapefruit" because its fruits were growing in clusters in the same manner as grapes.

According to early records, grapefruits were discovered in 18th century West Indies and the first planted grapefruit trees were in Florida in 1820.

For centuries grapefruit oil was used to reduce inflammation, sugar cravings, weight gain, and cure hangovers. It is a very versatile essential oil with a clean scent and a slightly bitter taste like the fruit. It has all the smell and taste that's unique to citrus fruits.

Studies have shown that grapefruit oil induces relaxation. People who use grapefruit oil report a reduction in the amount of stress they feel. It helps to reduce sugar cravings and increase weight loss. It relieves depression and fluid retention. Grapefruit oil helps the immune system to function properly and eliminates toxins.

The active compounds in grapefruit oil are Myrcene and D-Limonene. Direct sunlight should be avoided up to 12 hours after the external application of grapefruit oil. Also, see your physician before use if you're on any medication because it could interact with some drugs.

14. Helichrysum

The scientific name is *Helichrysum italicum.*

Helichrysum oil has been used by traditional Mediterranean medicine practitioners for centuries. It is usually called "The Everlasting Flower" because it is able to restore the skin to a healthy form and improve complexion. Helichrysum oil is among the best natural alternatives to costly facial serums and creams. Only a few drops of helichrysum will provide you with medicinal benefits without having to use harsh chemicals.

It is a medicinal plant that has natural antibiotic, antimicrobial and anti-fungal benefits. It is a special oil because it boosts the growth of neurological tissues. Helichrysum has over 500 species. The oil is gotten through steam distillation of the flowers and leaves which are the most important parts. Helichrysum has been found to have antimicrobial and anti-inflammatory properties.

It relieves symptoms of allergies. It helps to heal wounds, and relieve indigestion. It could also inhibit the growth of Candida and stop skin inflammation.

The active compounds are Italidone, Y-Curcumene, Neryl acetate, and L-Limonene.

15. Hyssop

The scientific name is *Hyssopus officinalis.*

Hyssop is a very uncommon oil with plenty of medicinal properties. For millennia, hyssop has worked as a purifying and cleansing agent.

Romans adored hyssop because of their belief that it helps to keep them safe from plagues. Because of that belief, many people dry hyssop and hang around their homes because they want to prevent "evil eye" or negativity. People sometimes leave it near graveside to secure the dead.

Hyssop was mentioned severally in the Bible. In the book of Leviticus, it was recorded that God directed his people to perform ceremonial cleansing with hyssop. In one record, God commands his priests to combine hyssop, scarlet yarn, and cedarwood with the blood of a clean bird to spray on a person who just recovered from skin illness.

The leaves of the plant are processed to extract the essential oil.

According to a study, hyssop oil is able to relax the muscles and could be a potential remedy for herpes type 2 virus.

Hyssop is an antibacterial, anti-inflammatory and antiviral. It reduces anxiety, helps in detoxification and keeps the mind alert. It also boosts the respiratory system.

The active compounds in hyssop oil are TransPinocamphone, Cispinocamphone, and Beta-Pinene. Hyssop oil should not be used when pregnant because it may induce contraction of the uterus. Also, not more than 30 drops of hyssop should be used daily.

16. Jasmine

The scientific name is *Jasminum grandiflorum*.

You are probably thinking of your neighbor's daughter named Jasmine. Jasmine is quite popular and fascinating. When Jasmine blooms at night, the atmosphere is filled with its alluring and unmistakable scent. Since it blooms only at night, it's fragrance is sweet, romantic and nice, a very common quality of flowers that bloom in the dark.

Jasmine is a very popular name for women in the Middle Eastern region and the Indian subcontinent even though people from other parts of the world bear the name. Romance and love stories have been told with Jasmine as the muse. Some poets have also used Jasmine as an inspiration for some of their poems.

The flowers of Jasmine are processed to extract the Jasmine essential oil. It has been known as a natural treatment to improve mood, get rid of stress and balance hormones.

Asians have used Jasmine oil for centuries as a natural remedy for depression, emotional stress, anxiety, insomnia, and low libido.

According to research, Jasmine oil can increase the rate of breathing, blood oxygen saturation, and diastolic and systolic blood pressure. Also, it improves the alertness of users and boosts their energy.

Jasmine oil is known for soothing PMS symptoms, cramps and menopausal symptoms. It is also an aphrodisiac and an anti-anxiety remedy. It relieves pain, stress and improves sleep.

The active compounds in Jasmine oil are Phytol, Benzyl acetate, Benzyl benzoate. Jasmine oil should not be used during pregnancy because it is an emmenagogue and can increase the flow of blood to the pelvic region.

17. Juniper Berry

The scientific name is *Juniperus communis*.

Juniper berry has been used as herbal medicine since the days of the Greek and Arabian physicians. It was used as an antiseptic during the bubonic plague when people hoarded a few berries in their mouth to prevent infection.

Surgeons also used juniper tea to disinfect their tools. In the past, Indians of the American plains made food from juniper berry. It might interest you to note that juniper berry is not even a berry, just a cone having unusually fleshy and merged scales that makes it look like a berry.

The plant's "berries" are processed through steam distillation to produce a sweet essential oil with a balsamic scent.

Juniper berry is useful in detoxification and boosting the immune system. The essential oil is often used as a natural remedy to treat respiratory problems, sore throats, muscle aches, arthritis, and fatigue.

Research has shown that juniper berry essential oil can be a natural anti-fungal and antibacterial agent. It detoxifies the body and treats skin conditions. It helps the digestive system and enhances the function of the immune system. The active compounds are Sabinene and Alpha-Pinene. Juniper berry oil should be diluted for people with sensitive skin before topical application.

18. Lemongrass

The scientific name is *Cymbopogon flexuosus.*

Most people can recognize lemongrass as a citrusy seasoning used by the Thais for cooking but only very few people know how much therapeutic power the grass possesses.

In traditional medicine, lemongrass and its oil have been used as a remedy for circulatory problems, menstrual irregularities, headaches, nervous system disorders, behavioral problems, and infections.

Some cultures often call it "fever grass" because it is able to make a fever go away. Its fever stopping activities are even boosted when it is mixed with black pepper oil.

In aromatherapy, lemongrass essential oil is used because it can be insect repelling, antibacterial, improve digestion, bring relief for muscle pain and body aches.

It is also used because of the flavor it adds to soups and teas.

The essential oil is extracted by steam distillation of the leaves, and it is fresh with a little lemon scent. Lemongrass essential oil provides a soothing, calming, balancing and stimulating effect.

Some studies show that lemongrass oil may reduce the symptoms of thrush in people with HIV/Aids.

Lemongrass is used mainly for its anti-fungal, anti-yeast and antibacterial properties. It reduces fever, boosts energy and enhances the function of the digestive system. It can relieve headaches and stomachaches and help the ligaments and tendons to function. The active compounds in lemongrass essential oil are Geranial, Geraniol, Neral farnesol.

Pregnant women are not advised to use it because the oil can trigger menstrual flow. It should be avoided by nursing mothers and children.

19. Lime

The scientific name is *Citrus aurantifolia*.

The origins of limes remain quite unclear because some people argue that it came from the Indonesian archipelago while others say it is a native of the mainland of Asia.

It is thought that around A.D. 1000, the Arabs might have carried lemons and limes from India to Africa and the eastern Mediterranean countries. The western Mediterranean countries got to know lime from the returning Crusaders in the 12th and 13th centuries.

When Columbus was making his second voyage to the West Indies in 1943, he carried some citrus fruit seeds, and he gave included limes. Before long, the trees were well distributed in Mexico, West Indies, and Florida.

Lime has a lot of uses as a food ingredient but it has even more therapeutic benefits. It clears the mind and improves the ability of the immune system to fight disease and cleanse the body.

The essential oil is gotten from the steam distillation of the entire lime peel.

Lime is useful for its antiseptic and antibacterial properties. It relieves some respiratory problems, stress, and anxiety. It is able to combat some skin conditions and boost hair growth. It improves mental clarity and is also a natural disinfectant. The active compounds in lime oil are Beta-cedrene, GammaTerpinene, Alpha-Pinenes, and D-Limonene. When using topically, do not stay in direct sunlight for about 12 hours after applying.

20. Manuka

The scientific name is *Leptospermum scoparium.*

According to legends Captain Cook and his crew arrived mercury Bay in 1769 with a crew infected with scurvy. The local Maori tribe of New Zealand welcomed him and kindly offered them a medicinal drink made with manuka leaves.

The Maori tribe has long cherished the manuka tree for its unique healing powers. They used the bark and leaves as a treatment for fever, colds, dysentery and some other skin ailments.

But now, manuka reminds people of honey, which is still very beneficial. The essential oil has several remedies. People around the world still use it as a plant-based remedy for a lot of skin problems like dermatitis, chronic sores, psoriasis, ringworm, eczema and athlete's foot.

The oil is used for healing and has anti-inflammatory, anti-fungal, and antibacterial properties. It is also a strong antioxidant. Often times people compare it's potency to that of tea tree oil but it is more suitable for sensitive skin because it is gentle and its scent is like honey and flowers. Manuka essential oil is extracted from the steam distillation of the manuka tree leaves.

Manuka oil is important because it reduces fever naturally, and combats infection. It is antiseptic and is a natural remedy for allergy symptoms, and skin irritations. It helps to induce relaxation and sleep. The active compounds in manuka essential oil are Cadena, PineneLeptospermone, Calamenene. The oil should not be used during pregnancy because it is spasmolytic, and therefore can induce muscle relaxation.

21. Marjoram

The scientific name is *Origanum majorana*.

The ancient Egyptians used marjoram for healing, preservation and disinfecting. It was said that Aphrodite, the goddess of love, had a fondling for this herb. Marjoram was known by the Greeks as "joy of the mountain" and they made wedding and funeral wreaths with it.

European women of the middle ages used marjoram as nosegays in a bouquet.

The essential oil is extracted from the steam distillation of the plant's leaves. The oil has a spicy and woody scent and produces a calming effect.

People often substitute marjoram for oregano because of their similar qualities but marjoram is milder with a finer texture. It releases a warming effect on the body and mind, strengthens the immune system and provides relief from muscle tension.

It is also a strong antibacterial and antiseptic agent.

From research, marjoram has been used to relieve arthritis, improve skin health and stimulate the immune system. Also, it enhances the function of the digestive system and respiratory system. It stops cramps and spasms and relaxes the mind and nerves.

The active compounds in marjoram oil are Alpha- & Y-Terpinenes, Linalool. Pregnant women should stay away from marjoram oil because it is an emmenagogue.

22. Melissa (Lemon Balm)

The scientific name is *Melissa officinalis*.

Melissa oil is not a popular essential oil but it has been used for therapeutic purposes for centuries. In the 14th century, the French Carmelite nuns included Melissa oil in the tonic water that they made. Melissa was called "The Elixir of Life" by a famous 16th-century philosopher, botanist, and physician named Paracelsus.

Melissa oil is part of the mint family. The oil is extracted by steam distillation of the flowers and leaves. Melissa oil is cherished for its antiviral, antibacterial, antidepressant, antispasmodic properties. It improves skin health and balance emotions. It prevents infection and improves mood.

Melissa oil is used for some respiratory troubles and also brings relief for PMS.

The active compounds are Citronellal, Geranial, Neral, Germacrene.

Melissa oil should not be used during pregnancy because it is an emmenagogue. Always dilute with a carrier oil before topical application on sensitive skin.

23. Myrrh

The scientific name is *Commiphora myrrha.*

Myrrh was found over 3,700 years ago. The ancient Egyptians used it to embalm their dead and as cosmetics and perfumes. From past records, myrrh is regarded as a valuable plant that it was sometimes as a wonderful natural antibiotic and it's therapeutic compounds have antifungal and antibacterial properties that can be used for a lot of health challenges. Oregano is useful in clearing allergy symptoms and boosting respiratory problems. It is an anti-inflammatory agent and has recently been found to be a potential anti-tumor agent. The active compounds in oregano oil are Thymol and carvacrol.

Oregano oil should not be used during pregnancy because it could be embryotoxic. Also, topical use may be followed by skin irritation, therefore the best approach is to dilute it with a carrier oil and then apply it on a small patch of skin to test it first. For internal use, oregano oil should not be used for more than ten consecutive days. There should be a one week break after using it for 10 days.

24. Roman Chamomile

The scientific name is *Chamaemelum nobile*.

Despite its name, Roman chamomile is not restricted only to the Romans as it is famous beyond ancient Rome. According to some discoveries, there are hieroglyphic records that show the cosmetic use of Roman chamomile for more than 2000 years. It was prescribed by early Greek physicians for its efficacy in treating female problems and fevers.

Roman chamomile has also been used by mothers as a skin ointment for their children because of its calming qualities.

Roman chamomile essential oil was used as medicine because it is antispasmodic. Nowadays, it is a natural remedy for anxiety, eczema, gout, heartburn, insomnia, and fever.

It is an antidepressant and also soothes hemorrhoids. It enhances the performance e of the digestive system and relieves arthritis.

The active compounds in Roman chamomile are Angelate, Esters, and Isobutyrate. Do not use Roman chamomile oil during pregnancy because it is an emmenagogue. Also, when used internally, it should be taken for two weeks at a time.

25. Spikenard

The scientific name is *Nardostachys jatamansi*.

Spikenard essential oil was one of the most precious and famous oils in the past. It was called "nard".

Apart from being mentioned in the Bible as the fragrance that that would be used in the symbolic marriage supper feast, spikenard was a major role player in Greek and Roman healing ceremonies. They also used it in cooking.

Spikenard is used in Ayurveda both for healing and creating a connection to the soul. Spikenard can be used to calm the nerves of people who suffer from anxiety.

It is also a great remedy for digestive issues, stress, infections, and insomnia.

Spikenard essential oil is extracted through steam distillation of the plant roots. The scent that comes from the oil is heavy, woody and sweet.

Spikenard protects the female reproductive system and boosts the immune system. It is an antibacterial, anti-inflammatory, and antifungal agent. It improves skin health. Spikenard also relaxes the mind and body and stops insomnia. The active compounds are Bornyl acetate, Valeranone, and AlphaPatchoulene. Spikenard should not be used during pregnancy because it triggers the uterus.

26. Turmeric

The scientific name is *Curcuma longa*.

Turmeric is currently famous for its use as a spice, medicine and coloring agent. However, turmeric did not get it's fame in these modern times as it has been used for 4,000 years by the Indians who practiced the Vedic culture. They used it both for cooking and for religious events. Turmeric is used in ayurvedic medicine to warm and strengthen the body.

During the middle ages, turmeric was known as Indian Saffron because of its orange-yellow color. To extract the essential oil, turmeric root is processed through steam distillation of the plant root. Turmeric has been adored for its potential anti-cancer properties. It also has antimicrobial, antibacterial, antiviral, antiallergic, antiparasitic, anti-fungal properties.

It boosts the digestive system and makes the liver healthy. As an anticonvulsant, it is able to avert seizures. Turmeric fights flu and cold and is also a remedy for anxiety and depression.

The active compounds are AlphaAtlantone, AlphaTurmerone, BetaTurmerone, Ar-Turmerone, and Curcumin.

When used topically, it is best to be cautious around fabrics because it may easily smudge the skin and clothes.

27. Vetiver

The scientific name is *Vetiveria zizanioides*.

Although it's native to India, many cultures have used vetiver essential oil for ages. The herb is widely used because people testify to its soothing, uplifting, shielding, and healing properties.

It is a sacred herb and the people of India and Sri Lanka refer to it as the "oil of tranquility".

People use it to make window blinds that can be used to prevent the intense heat. The vetiver is placed in the room and then the window blinds are sprinkled with water, this makes them emit the scent of the vetiver which in turn lowers the temperature of the air and body and keeps them cool.

The Javanese people used the root to weave mats and thatch for roofing their huts.

Vetiver essential oil is gotten from the steam distillation of the roots. The oil produces an earthy, sweet and smoky scent.

In the modern world, vetiver is used to treat some conditions like headaches, skin disorders, heatstroke, joint problems, and muscle aches. Vetiver oil also serves as an energy booster.

According to research, vetiver oil is a useful remedy for children with ADHD. Vetiver oil is useful for joint and muscle pain. It enhances cardiovascular health and improves neurological problems. It can also be anti-anxiety and improve focus.

The active compounds in vetiver oil are DeltaSelinene, BetaVetivenene, Khusimene. People with sensitive skin are advised to dilute with a carrier oil prior to topical application.

28. Wintergreen

The scientific name is *Gaultheria procumbens*.

Wintergreen is also known as "Nature's Aspirin". This plant has so many therapeutic properties and has been used as a remedy for several kinds of pain.

Wintergreen is used in Ayurveda to perform spiritual ceremonies based on the belief that the sacred plant could create a balance with its healing powers between the Earth and humans.

The native Americans used it as a remedy for musculoskeletal illnesses like arthritis. When the colonials visited America, they were taught about the plant by the native Americans.

The leaves of the wintergreen plant are processed by steam distillation to get wintergreen essential oil. The leaves are by default tasteless and odorless but after processing them and a certain compound they posses is disintegrated to methyl salicylate, then it begins to emit the minty aroma for which it is known.

According to research, wintergreen oil has antiarthritic, astringent, antiseptic, and analgesic properties.

The active compound in wintergreen oil is methyl salicylate and it is one of the most potent anti-inflammatory compounds in the world. Wintergreen is among the plants that have enough of the compound to be a natural reservoir.

Wintergreen oil is able to reduce headache, tension and muscle and joint pain. It enhances the function of the urinary system and makes PMS symptoms better. It serves as a remedy for respiratory conditions and can be used to lower swelling and irritation.

Wintergreen should not be taken internally because it contains methyl salicylate. The oil should be diluted before topical application.

29. Ylang Ylang

The scientific name is *Cananga adorata.*

People in the East and West have used ylang ylang for many purposes over the years. The Indonesians spread petals of ylang ylang flowers on the bed of couples before they consummate their wedding.

The Philippine healers used ylang ylang to make salves for treating cuts, insect bites, burns, scrapes, and snakebites.

Ylang ylang was used traditionally for centuries until it's medicinal properties were recognized by French chemists Rechler and Garnier at the start of the 20th century.

They found out that the oil was able to effectively treat a lot of diseases like typhus, malaria and intestinal infections. The chemists also found out that the oil was able to calm the heart in times of distress, and Ylang ylang oil is used in oriental medicine because of this effect.

The essential oil is extracted from the flower petals of the tree. It gives off a scent that is both flowery and sweet.

The meaning of Ylang ylang is "flower of flowers" and it got its name from its scent. The oil is known to be an antispasmodic, antidepressant and antiseptic.

The positive effect of ylang ylang on immune health makes it an amazing choice for treating disorders related to the digestive, endocrine, reproductive and cardiovascular systems.

Ylang ylang has been known to relieve stress and depression. Also, it reduces blood pressure and the heart rate of users.

The essential oil is used to improve skin health, improve libido and can reduce inflammation. The active compounds in ylang ylang are AlphaFarnesene, BetaCaryophyllene, Germacrene, Caryophyllene.

Ylang ylang should be used in low amounts because using it in excessive quantities may cause nausea, headache, and sensitivity.

Chapter Six

Remedial Uses of essential oils

1. Basil oil

❖ As an antibacterial and antifungal agent around the home.

Basil oil can be vaporized or diffused or even mixed with a natural cleaner. The mixture can be rubbed on surfaces and used to clear bacteria from bathrooms and kitchens.

❖ As a relief from flu and cold symptoms

Basil should be diffused in the home to prevent symptoms like congestion.

A steam bath should be prepared with 2 to 3 drops of basil oil. To open nasal passages, mix 2 drops of basil oil, together with a carrier and 2 drops of eucalyptus oil.

❖ As a remedy for Urinary Tract Infections

Dilute 1 to 2 drops of basil oil with a carrier oil or put 1 to 2 drops into food and consume internally. It detoxifies the urinary and digestive tracts.

❖ As a muscle relaxant

Use 3 drops of basil oil as a massage oil on painful, swollen joints or muscles to relax it. A bath water solution of Epsom salt, basil oil and lavender can be used to release tension in muscles.

❖ To reduce ear infection discomfort

Combine equal parts of frankincense oil, basil oil, and coconut oil. Rub behind the ears to stop swelling from an infected ear and help the healing

❖ Boost oral health

Put in some drops of pure basil oil in your toothpaste or mouthwash. This helps to keep your teeth and gum free from ulcers, viral blisters, toothaches, and sores.

❖ As an air freshener

Mix 4 to 6 drops of basil oil with baking soda. Use the mixture to clean kitchen appliances. Or, mix water, a few drops of basil oil and a natural cleaner together, then spray the mixture in the garbage can, toilet, and shower.

2. Bergamot oil

❖ To Improve mood and stop depression

Put 2 to 3 drops on your palms and cup your nose and mouth. Inhale slowly. Rub it on your feet and nape.

❖ Promote lymphatic drainage

Rub 2 to 3 drops of bergamot oil on your feet before you sleep. You can mix 3 to 5 drops with a carrier oil to make a massage oil that calms, relaxes and boosts lymphatic drainage.

❖ Enhances digestive system

Rub 3 to 5 drops on your stomach to improve digestion and monitor your appetite. This triggers the production of digestive juices and helps the intestinal muscles to contract.

❖ As a natural deodorant

Put some drops of bergamot oil in your deodorant or rub it directly on your armpits. Bergamot oil can be used together with cedarwood, sandalwood and lemon oils to create a unique fragrance

❖ To reduce stress and anxiety

Diffuse Bergamot oil in a room. Also, you can topically apply 1 to 2 drops on your wrists and temples to cope with stress.

❖ Deal with food cravings

Place in a diffuser and use in the home, at work or on the go to help deal with hunger pangs.

❖ Boost immunity

Bergamot can be consumed internally to combat pathogenic bacteria. You can also make a warm water bath with a few drops, diffuse it, or inhale it directly.

3. Birch oil

❖ Relief for spasms and muscle pain

Rub the oil on the affected area. 1 to 2 drops should be applied on the outside of the mouth to reduce toothaches.

❖ Relieve symptoms of Arthritis

Applying birch oil to the affected area can help reduce the pain of arthritis and rheumatism, and also boost circulation.

• As an anti-inflammatory

birch oil can help those who suffer from gout and reduce inflammation. 3 to 4 drops should be topically applied to the affected parts to reduce the pain.

❖ Treats ulcer pain and cramps

Mix 2 to 3 drops of birch oil with a carrier oil and rub it on the abdomen or, prepare a warm bath with 3 to 5 drops of the oil.

❖ To enhance mood and self-esteem

You can use birch oil to stimulate the nerves, circulatory and sensory systems because of its warming properties. Diffuse birch oil in the environment or rub it on your wrists, nape, and soles.

❖ Boost circulation

Apply birch oil to areas with poor blood flow to boost circulation.

❖ Detoxification of kidneys

Birch oil can remove toxins from the kidney by increasing perspiration and urination. Combine birch oil with a carrier oil. Massage the mixture all over your skin to help in detoxification of kidneys.

4. Black Pepper

❖ To Boost circulation

Prepare a warm compress and add 3 to 5 drops of black pepper oil on it, then place it on your abdomen or the affected area.

❖ To enhance digestion

For diarrhea, constipation, and gas, add 1 to 2 drops of black pepper oil to soup, smoothie or any dish you enjoy. You can also rub it on your abdomen.

❖ To relieve sprains and tendonitis

Apply topically to the affected area to lower muscle injuries and tendinitis.

❖ To relieve respiratory conditions

The oil can be inhaled or consumed internally. Rub 2 to 3 drops on your chest to open congested airways.

❖ To lower cigarette cravings

Inhaling or diffusing black pepper oil can help smokers to reduce their cravings.

❖ To soothe arthritis and rheumatism symptoms

Topical application on the affected area will soothe the symptoms of arthritis and rheumatism.

❖ Assists in detoxification

Black pepper can be used to lower inflammation and blood pressure and detoxify the body. Consume internally or rub 2 to 3 drops of black pepper oil to your soles.

5. Cardamom

❖ To relieve digestive issues

Cardamom oil can reduce the discomfort of intestinal diseases and lower symptoms of nausea, vomiting, and diarrhea. You can ingest 1 to 3 drops or rub directly on the abdomen.

❖ To Reduce Menstrual and PMS symptoms

Menstrual and PMS discomfort can be relieved by topical application of 3 to 4 drops of the oil on your abdomen.

❖ To improve sore throat

Cardamom is able to warm the body and trigger sweating to remove cough and congestion. Rub cardamom oil on your chest to clear the sore throat.

❖ As a natural aphrodisiac

Diffuse the oil or use 1 to 2 drops topically to improve arousal. It is a good remedy for loss of libido or frigidity, erectile dysfunction, and impotence.

❖ Reduce muscle pain and cramps

Cardamom has anti-inflammatory properties and can be used to improve symptoms of menstruation, arthritis, and menopause when applied to the affected area.

❖ To Reduce mental fatigue and brain fog

Topically apply 1 to 2 drops of cardamom oil on the nape of the neck.

❖ To freshen breath

Drop some cardamom oil into the water and shake in your mouth to stop bad breath and lower gum problems.

6. Cassia

❖ To Boost Healthy Blood Sugar Levels

Cassia can maintain blood sugar levels when ingested internally. Add 1 drop into coffee, tea, oatmeal or any warm and spicy meal.

❖ To Boost Metabolism

For a healthy body, 2 to 4 drops of cassia oil can be applied topically on the soles of your feet or abdomen to improve metabolism.

❖ To provide heat for cold extremities

Drop some cassia oil on the soles of your feet. Also, you can rub the oil on your legs or prepare a warm water bath with about 5 to 7 drops of oil. It would improve warmth in the body.

❖ To boost libido

Spread 2 drops of cassia oil on a handkerchief and cup it over your nose and mouth to inhale the scent.

❖ For lung detoxification

Inhale cassia oil spread over a handkerchief to help detoxify the lungs.

❖ Lower food cravings

Prepare a glass of water with 1 drop of cassia oil and 1 drop of lemon oil. The mixture will help enhance digestion and stop food cravings.

❖ To combat depression

Prepare a warm water bath with some drops of cassia oil.

7. Cedarwood

❖ To maintain focus and relieves symptoms of ADD/ADHD

Make a strong blend of cedarwood oil and take three deep inhalations of it for 30 consecutive days to improve ADHD symptoms.

❖ To clear acne and eczema

To naturally clear acne, combine 2 to 3 drops of the oil with a lotion and use it for a skin massage.

❖ To improve focus and boost concentration

Mix your skin lotion or soap with 2 to 3 drops of cedarwood oil. Also, you can diffuse it or directly sniff it in from the bottle.

❖ To relieve cough and sinus

Rub some quantity of cedarwood oil on the throat and chest to clear the respiratory tract and lungs.

❖ As an insect repellent

The topical application of cedarwood oil is able to prevent flies, mosquitoes and other insects. It can be mixed with water and used as a spray for couches and beds. Adding 3 drops of cedarwood oil to cotton balls placed in specific places in the house can prevent moths.

❖ To alleviate tension

Cedarwood can be inhaled directly, or applied topically or diffused to soothe the mind and release tight muscles.

❖ As an antifungal

Diffusing cedarwood oil or applying them on your body can help prevent internal and external fungal infections.

8. Cilantro

❖ To facilitate heavy metal detox

Consume 1 to 2 drops of cilantro oil at a time to eliminate heavy metal detox. Also, you can diffuse the oil.

❖ To boost liver function

For a healthy liver, 1 to 2 drops of cilantro oil can be added to food or drink. It can also be diffused or applied topically.

❖ To settle the abdomen

For relief, 3 to 5 drops should be applied topically to the stomach to relieve nausea and other stomach troubles.

❖ To boost anti-aging

Cilantro oil should be diffused around the home to help reduce oxidative stress and prevent the body from being damaged by free radicals.

❖ To maintain optimum blood sugar levels

Consume 1 to 3 drops of cilantro oil internally to assist and relieve diabetes naturally.

❖ Prevent cardiovascular disease

Swallow 1 drop of cilantro oil to protect your cardiovascular system from oxidative damage.

❖ To Prevent Urinary Tract Infection

Rubbing cilantro oil on your stomach or consuming it can release antibacterial compounds that prevent germs from clogging the urinary tract.

9. Cinnamon Bark

❖ To improve heart health

Prepare a mixture of 2 to 3 drops of cinnamon and ½ teaspoon of coconut oil. Rub the mixture on your chest to boost blood circulation and cleanse the arteries.

❖ To help keep the blood healthy

Cinnamon oil can be inhaled, topically applied to the wrists and chests or diffused to avoid overeating, moodiness and chronic fatigue.

❖ To reduce high cholesterol

Consume 1 to 2 drops of cinnamon oil to combat high cholesterol. Cinnamon oil reduces the activity of HMG CoA, the enzyme that synthesizes cholesterol in the body.

❖ To fight infections

Diffusing cinnamon oil daily can prevent infection or bring relief for a current infection.

❖ Enhance weight loss

Mix 1 to 2 drops of cinnamon bark oil to food, smoothies, fruit and other edibles to reduce the rate of entry of glucose into the blood.

❖ To combat parasites

Ingesting cinnamon oil can inhibit the growth of parasites in the body.

❖ To relieve sore throat

Prepare a hot drink made up of 1 drop of cinnamon oil, honey, and lemon water. Drink it every morning to relieve sore throat and also open nasal passages.

10. Citronella oil

❖ Insect repellent

Create a blend of coconut oil and 3 to 5 drops of citronella oil, then rub all over the body like a lotion. Or drop some of the oil in a water-filled spray bottle and use it as an insect repellent spray for your skin, furniture, and clothes.

❖ Stop swelling and pain

Use 3 to 5 drops of citronella oil to massage tissue, swollen joints, and muscles. Also, you can prepare a warm bath with 5 drops of citronella oil and soak in it.

❖ For body and mind relaxation

Diffusing citronella oil can activate its relaxing properties and reduce stress. Also, you can use citronella oil to massage the nape of your neck.

❖ For body and kidney detoxification

Drinking a mixture of 2 drops of citronella oil with a teaspoon of raw honey, hot water and 2 drops of lemon oil can increase urination and sweating to eliminate toxins.

❖ As a deodorant

Add citronella oil to a spray bottle and spray on appliances in the home to destroy bacteria and fungi.

❖ To improve hair health

Mix 5 to 7 drops of citronella oil with your conditioner or shampoo. Also, mix citronella oil with 1 teaspoon of coconut oil and massage into your scalp and hair.

11. Clary Sage

❖ To improve hormonal balance

Rub 3 drops of clary sage oil on your stomach, diffuse the oil or apply 2 drops on your neck region to monitor estrogen levels and improve the health of the uterus.

❖ To relieve menstrual discomfort

Consume internally or rub on your stomach to reduce some PMS symptoms.

❖ Boosts restfulness

To use the oil as a natural sedative against insomnia and anxiety, apply1 to 2 drops on the sole of your feet, your neck and diffuse it near your bed.

❖ To Promote healthy circulation

Apply the oil all over your chest and limbs to open up your blood vessels and lower blood pressure.

❖ To reduce cholesterol

Diffuse clary sage oil or prepare a warm water bath with 5 drops of the oil to lower cholesterol.

❖ To combat leukemia

Internal consumption of clary sage oil can induce apoptosis which aids in killing leukemia cell lines.

❖ To boost skin health

Apply a mixture of Clary sage oil and jojoba oil on my skin to reduce inflammation and remove rashes.

12. Clove

❖ To combat Candida

The anti-fungal properties of clove are as effective as nystatin, an antifungal drug. Mix about 1 drop of clove oil in edibles or in a capsule. This should be done for two weeks to stop Candida.

❖ Boost oral health

Apply a mixture of 1 to 2 drops with coconut oil to the area of concern. It helps to relieve dental discomfort.

❖ To fight parasite

Consume clove oil for about two weeks to remove parasites from the body. It could be taken either in capsules or mixed with a carrier oil.

❖ To block oxidative stress

Topical application of clove oil on your chest and neck helps to prevent slow aging by reducing the effects of free radicals. You can also diffuse it or use a carrier oil.

❖ To clear acne

To clear skin infections and acne, prepare a mixture of 3 drops of clove oil and 2 teaspoons of raw honey. Massage your face with the mixture and leave it for some minutes. Rinse your face and dry it.

❖ To combat cold and flu viruses

The topical application of clove oil or diffusion will help boost the immune system and increase the body's ability to fight disease.

❖ To maintain healthy blood pressure levels

Apply a mixture of clove oil and coconut oil to your wrists or diffuse the oil in your surroundings to reduce high blood pressure and ease stress.

13. Coriander

❖ To maintain healthy blood sugar levels

Swallow 1 drop of coriander oil when needed to help lower cholesterol and control blood sugar levels and blood pressure.

❖ Alleviate gas, nausea and bloating

Consume 1 drop of coriander oil internally or rub 2 to 3 drops on your stomach. It aids in relaxing the digestive system and reduce nausea causing irritation.

❖ To reduce skin irritation and rashes

Rub 2 to 3 drops of coriander oil to the affected area to relieve itchy skin and rashes.

❖ Relieve anxiety

To relax your mind, diffuse coriander oil around your house. Or prepare a blend of coriander, Roman chamomile and lavender, then rub the mixture on the nape of your neck and soles of your feet.

❖ To relief joint pain and muscle pain

Rub directly on the affected area to provide soothing relief to arthritis pain, rheumatism, and others.

❖ To soothe adrenal fatigue

Rub coriander oil on the soles of your feet or the nape of your neck to improve adrenals function.

❖ To boost appetite

Swallow one drop of coriander oil to improve appetite. You can also put 2 to 3 drops on your palms or handkerchief, then sniff it in for 5 minutes.

14. Cumin

❖ To enhance digestion

Add 1 drop of cumin oil to food to help the digestive system function effectively.

❖ To detoxify the body

Consume 1 drop of cumin oil internally to remove toxins from the body.

❖ To avoid infections

Prevent infections on internal and external cuts and wounds by ingesting 1 drop of cumin oil. Also, lace 2 to 3 drops of the oil and put it on the infection.

❖ To provide relief for cramps

The topical application of cumin oil to the affected area will help to stop cramps and spasms that result from digestion or menstruation.

❖ To tone body systems

Stimulate your body organs by preparing a mixture of 2 to 4 drops of cumin oil with 1 teaspoon of coconut oil and then massaging it onto the soles of your feet.

❖ To regulate the menstruation cycle

As an emmenagogue, cumin oil helps to regulate the menstrual cycle properly. To achieve this, do a deep inhalation from the bottle, rub it over your uterus or ingest it.

❖ To support nerve tissue

Diffuse cumin oil in your home or put 1 drop of cumin oil in your food to reduce nervous disorders.

15. Cypress

❖ Reduce the visibility of cellulite and varicose veins

Mix 2 to 4 drops of cypress oil to a carrier oil and apply to areas with veins and cellulite to boost blood flow.

❖ To reduce hemorrhoids

Rub 3 to 4 drops of cotton ball on the area of concern to reduce and avert hemorrhoids.

❖ To reduce restless leg syndrome

Rub cypress oil on the affected area to lower the discomfort connected to restless leg syndrome.

❖ To lower swelling from strains and sprains

The topical application of cypress oil to the affected area helps lower problems related to cramps and muscle strains.

❖ To improve prostate health

Prepare a bath with cypress oil, or use it in a massage blend to reduce the size of a swollen prostate. Also, you can visit a qualified and clinically trained aromatherapist to advise you on how to use it as a suppository.

❖ Relieves Edema and Fluid Retention

Topical application on the wrists, stomach, soles of the feet and nape of the neck is able to increase sweating which helps the body to remove toxins rapidly.

❖ To calm respiratory conditions

Prepare warm bath water with 5 drops of cypress oil. You can dilute the oil and use it as a vapor rub for your chest.

16. Eucalyptus oil

❖ To provide relief for symptoms of pneumonia and bronchitis

Prepare a homemade vapor rub with 3 to 5 drops of eucalyptus oil and equal amounts of coconut oil and peppermint oil. Apply the mixture topically on your chest to help blood vessel dilation and allow the flow of oxygen into the lungs.

❖ To reduce earaches

Drop some quantity of eucalyptus oil in a pot of boiling water. Bring the pot away from the heat, cushion your head with a towel and inhale the steam. You can also use the oil as a massage ointment for the skin beside your ear.

❖ To reduce asthma and allergies

The topical application of eucalyptus oil on the chest is able to reduce sinusitis and allergy symptoms. Also, you swish 1 to 2 drops of the oil in your mouth.

❖ To boost focus and energy

Diffuse eucalyptus oil around your home, office or surrounding to improve alertness and maintain focus. You can also apply some drops on your neck or temples.

❖ To reduce shingles

The topical application of eucalyptus oil to your skin will relieve you instantly from pain and itching related to shingles.

❖ To prevent infection of wounds

The topical application of eucalyptus oil to the affected area two times daily will release antiseptic properties and prevent infection of wounds.

17. Fennel oil

❖ To help digestion

Ingest 1 to 2 drops of fennel oil by preparing tea with it, adding it to water or putting it in a capsule. It helps to balance the ph level in the abdomen and reduce acid reflux.

❖ To improve colic

Fennel oil provides a safe way for breastfeeding mothers to reduce colic pain. Drinking fennel tea can reduce the pain and raise movement in the small intestine. Also, a drop of fennel oil can be diluted and topically applied to the baby's abdomen.

❖ To avoid edema and fluid retention

Make an ointment with 1 to 2 drops of fennel oil and equal amounts of grapefruit oil. Rubbing the ointment on the affected part can prevent fluid retention in the body.

❖ To alleviate PMS and Menstrual pain

Adding 1 to 2 drops of fennel oil to teach or water helps to reduce frequent contractions of the uterus. Rub the oil on your stomach to maintain a healthy menstrual cycle and improve female reproductive health.

❖ To alleviate menopausal symptoms

Ingesting fennel oil or rubbing it on the abdomen can help to avoid bone loss in those with osteoporosis as a result of menopause.

❖ To trigger breast milk production

Ingest some drops of fennel oil or make tea with it. This helps to boost the hormones that support breast milk.

❖ To reduce gas and bloating

Ingesting fennel oil can improve digestion and soothe hunger pangs.

18. Fir Needle oil

❖ To alleviate respiratory problems

Diffuse 5 drops of fir needle oil and inhale it. It helps to clear respiratory problems resulting from common cold and flu.

❖ To heal broken bones

Dilute fir needle oil with a carrier oil like coconut oil. Rub it on the area needing repair three times daily.

❖ To fix ligament tears

Heal ligament tears by rubbing fir needle oil on the problematic areas to hasten recovery.

❖ To reduce tumors

Ingest 1 to 2 drops or use the oil to massage the affected area as a supplement for reducing cancerous tumors.

❖ To relieve pain

Rub it on aching muscles and areas where you feel body aches to feel relief.

❖ To prevent osteoporosis

Combine fir essential oil with a carrier oil and apply to the affected area to assist in increasing bone density.

19. Frankincense oil

❖ To Assist cancer-fighting protocols

To assist in inhibiting some types of cancer cells, ingest 2 to 3 drops of frankincense oil, or use it to massage the affected area, or ask a physician to guide you in using it as a suppository.

❖ To relieve joint pain and inflammation

Use frankincense oil as a massage oil for parts of the body where there's joint or muscle pain.

❖ To enhance the immune system

Ingest frankincense oil, diffuse around the home or apply topically on the soles of the feet, wrists, and temples to boost the immune system.

❖ To promote relaxation

Diffuse frankincense oil around the home during meditation or use it as an anointing oil for the family to develop a relaxed feeling.

❖ To alleviate cold and flu symptoms

Apply topically 2 to 3 drops of frankincense oil on your chest or diffuse 5 drops of oil and inhale deeply for 5minutes.

❖ To lessen stretch marks and wrinkles

Combine 2 to 3 drops of frankincense oil with the same amount of jojoba or coconut oil and rub the mixture on the affected parts to reduce scars, stretch marks and wrinkles.

❖ To assist people with Alzheimer's and brain injury

To help improve the cognitive health of people having brain issues, ingest the oil, rub at the nape of the neck and under the nose or diffuse it.

20. Geranium

❖ To promote skin health

Geranium slows down the appearance of wrinkles and delays aging. Make a mixture of 2 drops of geranium oil to the same amount of coconut oil and use it two times daily.

❖ To maintain hormone levels

Combine 1 to 2 drops of geranium oil with some quantity of orange oil, clary sage oil, and carrier oil. Rub the mixture on your abdomen just before the start of your menstrual cycle

❖ To detoxify kidneys

Ingest geranium oil or apply topically on the stomach to remove toxins from the body.

❖ To boost muscle health

Mix 5 drops of geranium oil with 1 tablespoon of jojoba oil to make massage oil, then apply it on muscles and skin to tone and prevent sagging.

❖ To prevent eczema and psoriasis

Apply a mixture of geranium oil and Shea butter to damaged prevent dryness and flakiness.

❖ To activate blood clotting

Ingesting geranium or applying topically can help to hasten the formation of blood clots.

❖ To prevent Alzheimer's and dementia

Apply geranium oil topically on your wrists, nape of your neck and temples to avoid conditions that result in memory loss.

21. Ginger oil

❖ To stop nausea and morning sickness

Rub 1 to 2 drops of ginger essential oil on your abdomen or diffuse 2 to 3 drops home to stop nausea.

❖ To improve digestion

Dilute a few drops of ginger oil with a carrier oil and apply the mixture on your stomach, or put 1 drop to your food. Also, you can inhale ginger oil to stop indigestion.

❖ To heal infections

When using ginger oil for external infections, put 2 to 3 drops directly on the affected part. To relieve internal infections, put some drops in your food, water or food. Drop it in one at a time, and keep tasting after every drop to make sure you don't exceed your tolerance level.

❖ To ease colds and sore throat

Prepare a cup of green tea with 1 drop of oil and drink it twice daily to release symptoms of cold and cough.

❖ To lower inflammation and joint pain

Ingest 1 to 3 drops of ginger oil once daily to stop inflammation, and reduce pain. Also, you can put 2 drops of ginger oil to the affected part.

❖ To relieve anxiety

Diffuse 3 to 5 drops of ginger oil to suppress feelings of depression. Also, you can prepare a warm water bath with 5 drops of oil.

❖ To relieve pain from strains and sprains

Put some quantity of ginger oil to the affected part or prepare a warm water bath with ginger oil to treat muscle and joint pain.

22. Grapefruit oil

❖ To improve weight loss

Diffuse a mixture of grapefruit oil and patchouli to improve your metabolism and lower appetite. Alternatively, you can put 2 drops in water, a smoothie or any other edible liquid. Also, when you have food cravings, you can use the oil to massage your wrists and chests.

❖ To control weight loss

Put some drops of grapefruit oil and coconut oil to a cotton ball. You can rub it on your neck, wrists, and chest or even inhale the cotton ball to stop cravings.

❖ To improve lymphatic drainage

Ingest 1 to 2 drops of grapefruit oil or rub it directly over your kidneys to help remove toxins and salt.

❖ To improve gallbladder function and fat digestion

Use grapefruit, jojoba, and coconut oil to prepare a massage lotion. Rub it directly on your abdomen to detoxify and help with digestion.

❖ To fight candida

Ingest 1 to 2 drops of grapefruit oil or diffuse five drops to fight yeast and bacteria.

❖ To reduce cellulite

Combine grapefruit oil and coconut oil to make an ointment, then rub it on the affected areas daily to increase blood flow and lower inflammation.

23. Helichrysum oil

❖ To relieve nerve pain

Put two drops of helichrysum oil and frankincense oil on your wrists, temples and the soles of your feet daily. Do it for three weeks to boost your neurological system. Take a one week break then continue the cycle.

❖ To reduce bruising and bleeding

Topically apply 2 to 3 drops of helichrysum oil to the nape of your neck or any other place where you feel pain as many times as you desire each day.

❖ To reduce wrinkles

Mix 2 to 3 drops of helichrysum oil with a carrier oil and apply topically to areas that are more vulnerable to wrinkles.

❖ To aid digestion

Ingest helichrysum oil or rub it on your stomach to enhance secretion of gastric juices which aids digestion.

❖ To detoxify the liver and kidney

Ingest helichrysum oil to improve liver health and detoxify the blood.

❖ To inhibit cancer cell growth

Consume internally by putting some drops in a cup of tea to a glass of water to inhibit cancer tumor growth and protect cells from damage or death.

❖ To enhance the immune system

Diffuse the oil around you or ingest it to boost your immunity and gut health.

24. Hyssop oil

❖ To soothe respiratory conditions

Put 2 to 3 drops of hyssop oil in your tea, or rub it on your chest and throat to ease spasms in the respiratory system and relieve cough.

❖ To prevent infection

Hyssop can be used to prevent wounds and cuts from being infected. Put some drops of hyssop oil on the affected area.

❖ To fight parasites

Consume hyssop oil internally to remove internal parasites like flukes, hookworms, and tapeworms.

❖ To boost healthy circulation

Put hyssop oil in your tea or in hot water. Drink it to help proper blood circulation.

❖ To lower muscle pain and spasms

Prepare a warm water bath with Epsom salts and 5 to 10 drops of hyssop oil or apply 3 to 5 drops on the affected area to relax the muscles and prevent cramps.

❖ To improve the immune system

Drink tea or hot water that had been added hyssop oil to boost the immune system.

❖ To enhance skin health

Mix 2 to 3 drops of hyssop oil with a carrier oil and use it to massage the affected area. It helps to promote the growth of new cells and skin.

25. Jasmine oil

❖ To use as an aphrodisiac

Apply 5 drops of Jasmine oil topically on the soles of your feet, wrist or diffuse it in the home. It helps to enhance the physical signs of arousal.

❖ To fight anxiety and depression

Put 1 to 3 drops of Jasmine oil topically on your wrists, the nape of your neck, temples and the soles of your feet. It helps to enhance mood and increase energy levels.

❖ To combat wrinkles and aging skin

Combat wrinkles by adding 1 to 3 drops of Jasmine oil into your fave wash, lip balms, and lotion. It helps to maintain the radiance of the skin.

❖ To improve sleep

Diffuse Jasmine oil in the home or make a mixture with other essential oils like lavender and frankincense. Apply the mixture on your body to induce sedation and boost sleep.

❖ To maintain hormone balance

Apply jasmine oil topically or diffuse to help relieve PMS symptoms.

❖ To improve mood

Mix 1 to 2 drops of Jasmine oil with a carrier oil and apply on your wrists. Its warm, flowery scent helps to lift the spirit.

26. Juniper Berry oil

❖ To boost improve skin health

Put 1 or 2 drops of juniper berry oil to body or face wash to treat skin conditions. Alternatively, you can use 2 to 3 drops of the oil diluted with a carrier oil to rub the affected areas.

❖ To support the detoxification of the liver

Use juniper berry oil as a natural digestive to enhance nutrient absorption. Put some drops of juniper berry oil into a glass of water or a smoothie.

❖ To improve kidney and urinary health

Rub 1 to 3 drops of oil on your stomach or ingest it. It helps to improve urination and remove wastes from the digestive tract.

❖ To reduce bloating and gas

Use 1 to 3 drops of oil on your stomach or consume internally to remove excess fluids from the urethra and bladder which helps to lower gas and bloating.

❖ To improve sleep

Rub 1 to 3 drops of the oil on the soles of your feet, your chest, and your neck. Also, diffuse 5 drops before you sleep to avoid restlessness and help you sleep better.

❖ To relieve sore muscles

Massage juniper berry oil into the affected area to lower muscle pain and inflammation. You can also add it to bath water with Epsom salts and lavender oil.

27. Lavender oil

❖ To encourage good sleep

Lavender oil helps you sleep better when you diffuse 5 drops of it near your bed. You can also put 2 to 3 drops of the oil at the nape of your neck, your temples, and chest.

❖ To soothe burns, cuts, and sunburns

Apply a mixture of lavender oil and coconut oil to the affected area twice daily.

❖ To heal anxiety and stress

Prepare a warm water bath with lavender oil to help you relax. You can also diffuse it in your home or apply on the soles of your feet, wrists, and temple.

❖ To fight high blood pressure

Lavender oil can help you lower stress and maintain healthy blood pressure. You can diffuse in your home or around you as you carry out your day.

❖ To maintain healthy blood sugar balance

Put 1 drop of lavender oil to a cup of tea or a glass of water to reduce blood glucose. Alternatively, rub it on the nape of your neck, or diffuse it.

❖ To soothe headaches and migraines

Apply a mixture of 2 drops of lavender oil and 2 drops of peppermint oil on the nape of your neck to release tension and relieve pain. You can also inhale lavender oil for 15 minutes.

❖ To improve skin health

Apply lavender oil topically or combine with coconut oil for sensitive skin. Also, you can mix lavender oil with frankincense oil to improve skin health.

28. Lemon oil

❖ To promote lymphatic drainage

Put 1 to 2 drops directly on your lymph nodes to reduce swelling. You can also diffuse it.

❖ To remove mucus and phlegm

You can relieve congestion by direct inhalation of lemon oil. Alternatively, mix it with a carrier oil and rub it on your nose and chest.

❖ To enhance mood

Rub lemon oil on your wrists and chest to improve your mood. Alternatively, diffuse it around you.

❖ To aid gallbladder health and removal of gallstone

Create a mixture with 10 drops of lemon oil, 1 quart of sauerkraut juice, 10 drops of peppermint oil, and 1 quart of tomato juice.

Share the mixture equally into two jars. Drink the two jars on two consecutive days.

❖ To improve the immune system

Ingest lemon oil internally to remove pathogenic organisms that cause illness in the body.

❖ To reduce symptoms of allergy

Mix 1 to 2 drops of lemon oil with equal amounts of lavender and peppermint to fight allergy symptoms.

29. Lemongrass oil

❖ To repel bugs

Make a bug spray with 10 to 15 drops of water or diffuse it around the house to prevent insects. It can also repel fleas from the coat of insects by rubbing the coat with 5 drops of lemon oil.

❖ To boost skin health

Make your skin glow by adding lemongrass oil to soaps, lotions, shampoos, deodorants abs conditioners.

❖ To treat gastric ulcers

Prepare soup, tea or smoothie with lemongrass oil or infused lemongrass water to relieve stomach distress.

❖ As a natural deodorizer

Make an air freshener by mixing 5 to 10 drops of lemongrass oil with water. Or, diffuse it in the home. You can add other oils to customize the fragrance like lavender or peppermint oils.

❖ To reduce fever

Taking lemongrass oil internally is able to reduce symptoms of fever.

❖ To reduce cholesterol consumption

Consume 1 to 2 drops of lemongrass in a glass of water or a capsule to reduce cholesterol in the body.

❖ To treat candida/yeast infection

Ingest 1 to 2 drops of lemongrass oil.

30. Lime oil

❖ To relieve sore throat

Consume lime oil internally by placing 1 to 2 drops of the oil under your tongue. Or rub 2 to 4 drops of lime oil mixed with peppermint on your throat.

❖ To purify water

Put in a few drops of lime oil to 8 ounces of water before drinking. It removes bacteria in water and boosts internal and external bacterial infections.

❖ To cultivate lymphatic drainage

Combine lime oil, coconut oil, Rosemary oil, and geranium oil. Rub the mixture directly on your lymphatic pathways to remove wastes.

❖ To improve gallbladder function and digestion of fat

Prepare bath water or compress with a mixture of lime oil, rosemary oil, lemon oil, and carrier oil. Use it to massage your gallbladder.

❖ To improve mood and maintain balance

Prepare a warm water bath with 5 to 10 drops of lime oil to reduce stress and anxiety. Also rub it on your temples, stomach, the soles of your feet and the nape of your neck.

❖ To heal skin conditions

Dilute lime oil with jojoba oil or coconut oil. Rub the mixture on the affected area twice daily to relieve some skin conditions.

31. Manuka

❖ To heal acne, psoriasis, and eczema

Mix manuka oil with Shea butter and honey to make a mild cream. Rub on your skin to remove acne.

❖ To soothe allergy symptoms

Rub Manuka oil on the parts of your skin that are easily triggered by allergens. You can also diffuse 6 to 8 drops of manuka oil around you to calm allergic reactions.

❖ To remove scars and reduce age spots

Put some drops of manuka oil on a face or body lotion to help in rejuvenating damaged skin.

❖ To help relaxation and sleep

Diffuse manuka around you in your home, your bedside and your home to improve your sleep.

❖ To heal athlete's foot

Put 6 drops of manuka oil into warm water to make a foot soak. Soak your feet in the mixture for 20 minutes daily.

❖ To soothe respiratory conditions

Mix 6 to 8 drops of manuka oil into boiling water and inhale the vapor for 5 minutes. Or diffuse it in the home to relieve respiratory conditions.

❖ To promote oral health

Ingest manuka oil to heal gum and tooth disease.

32. Marjoram oil

❖ To relieve gastric ulcers

Consume 1 to 2 drops of marjoram internally to relieve symptoms of gastric ulcers. You can also use it to make tea.

❖ To alleviate headaches, back pain, and neck pain

Rub marjoram oil on the areas where you feel the pain to relax your tense muscles.

❖ To stop muscle pain and spasms

Dilute 3 to 5 drops of marjoram oil and apply it to the affected area two times daily to relieve pain from inflammation, fever, cold and toothache.

❖ To prevent infection

Topical application of 2 to 5 drops of marjoram oil will help to prevent illnesses and infections.

❖ To reduce stress and anxiety

Dilute marjoram oil and apply topically on your wrists and the nape of your neck. Also, direct inhalation from the bottle or diffusion is another way of using marjoram oil for its sedative properties.

❖ To relieve stomach cramps and flatulence

The oil has sedative properties that relax the digestive system.

Ingest marjoram oil by putting 1 drop under your tongue. For topical application, dilute it and rub it on your lower back and abdomen.

❖ To regulate blood pressure

Consume internally by putting marjoram oil under your tongue. For topical application, apply diluted marjoram oil over your heart.

33. Rose oil

❖ To fight depression

Make a mixture of rose oil with lavender oil. You can either diffuse it or rub 1 to 2 drops of the mixture on the nape of your neck or your wrists.

❖ To enhance libido

Diffuse rose oil in your home to treat sexual dysfunction. You can also rub 2 to 3 drops of rose oil on your neck and chest.

❖ To improve skin health

Add rose oil to body wash, face wash, or lotion to treat skin conditions or rub it directly on your skin.

❖ To support digestion

Rub 2 to 3 drops of rose essential oil on your stomach to relieve stomachaches.

❖ To relieve PMS and Menstrual Symptoms

Apply rose oil on your stomach or diffuse it in the home to relieve PMS and menstruation cramps.

❖ To alleviate seizures

Apply rose oil on the nape of your neck or your wrists or diffuse it to help with your seizures.

34. Orange oil

❖ To boost immunity

Ingest 1 to 2 drops of orange oil either by dropping it under your tongue or adding it to your favorite beverage or water.

❖ To help prevent cancer

Add 1 to 2 drops of oil into water or any beverage you like to prevent the growth of cancer cells.

❖ To encourage lymphatic drainage

Mix 2 to 4 drops of orange oil with coconut oil. Rub the mixture on your chest, lymph nodes, and lymphatic pathways.

❖ To fight anxiety

Add some drops of orange oil to your body wash, or diffuse it or inhale it directly to lower anxiety and stress.

❖ To improve mood

Apply orange oil on your skin or diffuse it to calm your body.

❖ To support digestion

Rub 2 to 3 drops of orange oil on your stomach area to improve digestion.

❖ To enhance detoxification

Ingest 1 to 2 drops of orange oil to reduce urine production.

35. Tea tree (melaleuca)

❖ To treat acne

Make your own face wash with 5 drops of tea tree oil and 2 teaspoons of raw honey. The mixture is just as effective as benzoyl peroxide but it has no side effects.

❖ To relieve dandruff

Create a shampoo with 5 to 10 drops of tea tree oil, coconut milk, aloe vera gel, and lavender oil. Or, put 5 drops of tea tree oil in your shampoo or conditioner to treat head lice and calm dry skin.

❖ To disinfect the home

Make a mixture of tea tree oil, vinegar, lemon oil, and water. Pit in in a spray bottle and use it for showers, kitchen appliances, sinks, and toilets.

❖ To heal psoriasis and eczema

Prepare a soothing and anti-inflammatory lotion by mixing 5 drops of tea tree oil, 1 teaspoon of coconut oil and 5 drops of lavender oil. Rub it on your skin two times daily.

❖ To relieve toenail fungus

Apply tea tree oil to the affected area to kill fungi causing ringworm, and athlete's foot. For severe fungi, combine tea tree oil with oregano oil.

❖ To clean infection and cut

Make an ointment with 2 drops of tea tree oil and 2 drops of lavender oil. Rub the mixture directly on the affected part to heal cuts, burns, and wounds.

36. Peppermint oil

❖ To relieve muscle pain

Apply 2 to 4 drops of diluted peppermint oil to the affected area to soothe the pain and calm muscles.

❖ To soothe respiratory conditions

Apply 2 to 4 drops of diluted peppermint oil to your chest and the nape of your neck. You can also put 10 drops in a pan of boiling water, cushion your head with a towel and inhale the aroma for about 5 minutes.

❖ To enhance energy

Direct inhalation of peppermint oil can bring a fast energy boost. You can also rub it on the nape of the neck, wrists, or temple or diffuse it to fight fatigue.

❖ To lower symptoms of allergy

Direct inhalation of peppermint oil or application of 2 to 3 drops of diluted peppermint oil on your neck, chest, and forehead.

❖ To relieve headache

Rub peppermint oil on your forehead and temples to open up your nasal passages when you have a sinus headache.

❖ To ease digestive conditions

Rub peppermint oil on your abdomen, ingest 1 to 2 drops or diffuse it to provide a remedy for bloating and nausea.

❖ To freshen your breath and combat cavities

Put one drop of peppermint oil in your mouthwash or toothpaste or drop the oil under your tongue, then drink some water.

37. Rosemary oil

❖ To enhance hair growth

Put 5 to 10 drops of Rosemary oil to shampoo or conditioner. Rub 3 to 5 drops of Rosemary oil in your scalp. Rinse it off after 5 minutes.

❖ To boost memory

Put some oil under your nose or on your forehead to improve alertness and enhance memory. You can also diffuse it in your home.

❖ To treat diabetes naturally

Put 1 to 2 drops of Rosemary oil in a glass of water. Drink it to supplement your body's sugar balance.

❖ To reduce pain

make an ointment with 2 drops of Rosemary oil, 1 teaspoon of coconut oil and 2 drops of peppermint oil. Massage it on your painful joints and muscles.

❖ To boost liver detoxification and gallbladder function

Make an ointment with 3 drops of Rosemary oil and ¼ teaspoon of coconut oil. Apply it on your gallbladder two times daily to prevent the buildup of toxins.

❖ To detoxify the body

Rub 2 to 3 drops of Rosemary oil on your stomach to improve nutrient absorption. Also, consume internally.

❖ To combat respiratory issues

Diffusing Rosemary oil or rubbing it on your chest will help to remove mucus and soothe other symptoms of respiratory infections.

38. Patchouli

❖ To ease anxiety and depression

Prepare a warm water bath with 5 to 10 drops of patchouli oil or diffuse 5 drops of patchouli oil to help ease anxiety and depression.

❖ To lower inflammation

Massage your stomach, feet, lower back and other inflamed areas with 3 to 5 drops of patchouli oil.

❖ To fight infection

Prepare a warm water bath with patchouli oil to keep wounds from being infected. Also, you can place the oil directly on the wound.

❖ To Help erectile dysfunction

Put 1 to 3 drops of patchouli oil on the nape of your neck, temples and the soles of your feet to help people with impotence. Or, diffuse 5 drops around your home.

❖ To vitalize skin and hair

For hair growth, massage your scalp with patchouli oil or mix it with your conditioner.

For rejuvenating skin, mix patchouli oil, jojoba oil or coconut oil. Rub the mixture on your face or add it to your face lotion or face wash.

❖ To repel insect

Fill a spray bottle with water and 5 to 10 drops of patchouli oil. Spray it on your skin, clothes, furniture or sheets to keep insects away.

39. Melissa oil

❖ To prevent dementia

Diffuse Melissa oil daily to help prevent the start of dementia.

❖ To treat eczema

Prepare a mixture of 5 drops of Melissa oil and 1 ounce of carrier oil. Use it on your face for acne and eczema. You can also add it to moisturizer, or make a spray solution and spritz on your face daily.

❖ To heal cold sores and herpes

Rub 2 to 3 drops of diluted Melissa oil on the affected area to treat herpes virus and cold sores.

❖ To improve hypoglycemia

Ingest a few drops to maintain glucose levels at a healthy level.

❖ To relieve feelings of depression and anxiety

Rub Melissa on your ears, wrists and the nape of your neck. Also, diffuse it to feel peace and warmth.

❖ To reduce vertigo and nervousness

Rub 2 to 3 drops of Melissa oil to the nape of your neck, and your ears to stop nervousness. You can also consume internally by putting 1 drop of Melissa oil to tea or water.

❖ To maintain healthy blood pressure

Relieve hypertension and keep blood pressure levels low, ingest 1 to 2 drops or rub it on your chest or the nape of your neck.

40. Myrrh

❖ To reduce inflammation

Use a cold compress to massage 2 to 3 drops of myrrh oil to the inflamed area to stop swelling and avoid infections.

❖ To treat vaginal and oral yeast

Ingest 1 drop of myrrh oil, rub 2 or 3 drops of myrrh oil mixed with a carrier oil on the affected parts.

Oral thrush can be relieved with gargling natural mouthwash and 1 to 2 drops of myrrh oil many times a day.

❖ To relieve gum disease and mouth infections

Use myrrh oil together with your toothpaste and mouthwash to avoid gum disease and mouth infections.

❖ To combat parasite and fungal infection

Apply topically on the site of infection or ingest 1 to 2 drops of oil in a capsule or with water.

❖ To fight cancer

Applying myrrh oil directly to a skin cancer site two times daily can help to provide anti-cancer benefits.

❖ To treat wounds and ulcers

Dilute 2 to 3 drops of myrrh oil with a carrier oil and rub it on the affected area two times a day to boost white blood cells.

41. Oregano

❖ To inhibit bacteria

Apply oregano oil diluted with a carrier oil on the soles of your feet or ingest it for 10 consecutive days and then take a break before you repeat the cycle.

❖ To combat Candida and fungal overgrowth

The topical application of oregano can heal toenail fungus. Also taking 2 to 4 drops of oregano oil two times daily for 10 days helps treat yeast and fungi.

❖ To combat bronchitis and pneumonia

Rub 2 to 3 drops of diluted oregano oil on external infections. To inhibit internal bacteria, consume 2 to 4 drops of oregano oil two times daily for 10 consecutive days.

❖ To stop MRSA and Staph infection

Ingest 3 drops of oregano oil with a carrier oil either in a capsule, or your favorite food or drink twice daily for 10 days to inhibit MRSA.

❖ To fight parasites and intestinal worms

Ingest oregano oil for 10 days at a stretch to fight parasites.

❖ To remove warts

Mix oregano oil with another essential oil or clay to help reduce and remove warts.

42. Roman chamomile

❖ To fight anxiety and depression

Inhale Roman chamomile directly from the bottle or diffuse 5 drops to help reduce stress and stops relaxation.

❖ To improve digestion and leaky gut

Rub 2 to 4 drops of Roman chamomile on the stomach to stop various gastrointestinal disturbances. Children who have colic and diarrhea should be given low doses.

❖ To boost restful sleep

Inhale Roman chamomile directly from the bottle, rub on the temples or diffuse at your bedside to combat insomnia and get a night of healthy sleep.

❖ To Soothe Children

Diffuse the oil around or rub it on the skin of children to stop them from crying and reduce earaches, fevers and other children's problems. Even children with ADD/ADHD get relief from Roman chamomile.

❖ To improve skin health

Soak up 2 to 3 drops of Roman chamomile with a cotton ball and rub on the affected area or mix 5 drops to a face wash to fight skin conditions and promote healthy skin.

❖ To improve heart health

Rub 2 to 4 drops of oil over your heart or ingest it by dropping some quantity of the oil under your tongue.

❖ To relieve nausea

Inhale Roman chamomile from the bottle or mix it with lavender, ginger, and peppermint oils to calm nausea. You can also apply it directly to your temples or diffuse it.

43. Spikenard oil

❖ To treat a bacterial infection

Ingest 1 to 2 drops of spikenard oil to heal internal infection or rub 3 to 5 drops on the affected area.

❖ To lower inflammation

Ingest 1 drop of spikenard oil every day or rub 3 to 5 drops on your skin twice daily to reduce inflammation which could trigger other diseases. You can also diffuse the oil in your home.

❖ To reduce anxiety and stress

Apply spikenard oil on the skin or diffuse it to soothe the mind.

❖ To improve the immune system

Rub spikenard oil on the nape of your neck or the soles of your feet to improve the immune system.

❖ To boost hair growth

Massage a mixture of 5 drops of spikenard oil with 1 teaspoon of coconut oil into your scalp. Rinse after 5 minutes. Or put 5 to 10 drops of spikenard oil into conditioner or shampoo.

❖ To relieve insomnia

Diffuse spikenard oil or rub 2 to 3 drops of oil on the nape of your neck or your temples.

❖ To heal constipation

Rub spikenard oil on your abdomen and the soles of your feet to stimulate the digestive system.

44. Turmeric

❖ To relieve joint pain and arthritis

Put some drops of turmeric oil on the affected part to relieve arthritis and pain.

❖ To improve digestion

Mix turmeric oil with a carrier oil and apply it on your stomach to lower symptoms of digestive conditions. You can also put 1 drop of oil in your favorite beverage.

❖ To fight cancer

Ingest 1 drop of turmeric oil mixed with food or beverage, in the morning and evening to supplement cancer medications. Alternatively, add this oil to a culinary carrier then take it internally in a capsule.

❖ To combat neurologic diseases

Consume turmeric oil internally, diffuse it or rub it on your skin to improve diseases like stroke and spinal cord injury.

❖ To relieve depression and anxiety

Diffuse turmeric oil in your surroundings throughout the day to boost mood and reduce depression.

❖ To help with epilepsy

Ingest 1 to 2 drops of turmeric oil to prevent seizures or drink hot turmeric tea frequently.

❖ To detoxify liver

Ingest turmeric oil or rub it on your skin to promote liver detoxification.

45. Vetiver

❖ To combat insomnia

Prepare a warm bath with vetiver oil and soak yourself for some minutes before bedtime. Or you can diffuse it at your bedside and inhale directly.

❖ To assist study and concentration

Diffuse vetiver oil near you while you study for your exams or work late in the night to help increase concentration and clear your thoughts.

❖ To combat aging and free radical damage

Apply vetiver oil on your skin or diffuse it to help slow aging and enhance skin health.

❖ To encourage scar healing

Rub 2 to 4 drops of vetiver oil on the affected area to rejuvenate skin and remove scars.

❖ To relieve people with ADD/ADHD

Diffuse a mixture of 2 drops of vetiver oil and 2 drops of lavender oil or spread it on the skin relax and calm children with ADD and ADHD.

❖ To improve Nervous tremors

Put 2 to 3 drops of oil on the nape of your neck or the soles of your feet or diffuse 5 drops to lower Parkinson's related tremors.

❖ To calm anxiety and nervousness

Soak yourself in a warm water bath mixed with vetiver oil, diffuse it or rub it on the skin to enhance relaxation and alleviate emotional stress.

46. Wintergreen

❖ To fight joint and muscle pain

Mix 3 to 5 drops of wintergreen oil with the same quantity of carrier oil and apply to the affected area to reduce irritation and pain around painful tissues and muscles.

❖ To enhance respiratory conditions

Mix 1 to 3 drops wintergreen oil with coconut oil. Massage the mixture on your chest and upper back to clear nasal passages.

❖ To combat and prevent infections

Apply diluted wintergreen oil topically or make a spray solution with 5 to 10 drops of oil and use it on your furniture, clothes and any hard surface. It inhibits the growth of fungi, bacteria, and viruses because of its disinfectant and antiseptic properties.

❖ To relieve gout symptoms

Apply a mixture of wintergreen oil with coconut oil to hasten the removal of toxins from the kidney.

❖ To boost skin health

Put 1 to 2 drops of wintergreen oil to a face wash or rub it on the affected area to improve skin health

❖ To fight fatigue

Before a workout, inhale wintergreen oil from the bottle or apply diluted oil to your wrist, chest, and neck to avoid drowsiness, boost stamina and increase alertness.

47. Ylang ylang oil

❖ To regulate blood pressure

Apply 1 drop of diluted ylang ylang oil over your heart or put 2 drops in a cup of warm tea or a cup of water to calm blood pressure.

❖ To promote skin health

Mix 2 drops of ylang ylang oil with the same quantity of jojoba oil or coconut oil. Rub it on the affected area twice daily to stop the skin from aging.

❖ To enhance mood and energy

Massage 3 to 5 drops of ylang ylang oil with a carrier oil on your temples and the back of your neck to improve your mood and treat mild depression.

❖ To balance hormones

Create an ointment with 2 drops of ylang ylang oil and 2 drops of lavender, then rub it on your lower belly and the nape of your neck.

❖ To lower frustration and anger

Inhale the oil from the bottle or diffuse it to help remove negative emotions.

❖ To improve self-confidence

Direct inhalation or topical application on the nape of your neck will help to improve your self-confidence.

❖ To improve libido

Rub ylang ylang oil on your wrists, temples and the nape of your neck or diffuse it to induce relaxation and boost the libido of men and women.

Chapter Seven

Essential Oils For Beauty And Skin

Life has many pleasures which we are often guilty of overlooking. It is not something we do consciously but it happens because we are caught up with other distractions.

We are also guilty of overlooking a lot of things when it comes to our skin. We shop for the best makeup products we can find but fail to notice the key things that make up a good skincare routine.

Essential oils are what we need to achieve healthy skin. This is the knowledge that the ancient people applied to maintain their beauty. Well, I'll let you know the essential oils that are amazing for skin care and why they are the best.

Essential oils play five roles when it comes to skin health.

1. They are effective in combating acne

2. They have antifungal properties

3. They are antioxidants and protect the skin from free radicals.

4. They have anti-aging benefits

5. They reduce inflammation

How To Use Essential Oils For Skincare

When using essential oils to improve skin health, there are two ways you can do it:

Use It As A Face Oil: Mix your essential oil with any carrier oil and apply directly on your face or, use water to dilute it before applying.

Combine With Your Face Mask: Put a few drops of essential oil in the routine face mask you already use.

There are lots of essential oils to choose from. But it is quite impossible to use all of them. Our best bet will be to choose the kind of oil that will soothe our skin type. This list of essential oil will help you know the best oils to use in your skincare routine.

The best oils for maintaining healthy skin

1. Tea Tree Oil: For blocking breakouts

The antimicrobial properties of tea tree oil make it very beneficial for combating acne. It is able to inhibit the growth of the acne-causing bacteria P. acne. It also clears the skin and prevents future breakouts.

To use tea tree oil for skin care:

Ingredients

5-6 drops of tea tree oil

A teaspoon of honey

Procedure

Make a mixture of tea tree oil and honey. Rub it on your face and let it sit for about 15-20 minutes before washing off. Do this once daily.

2. Lavender oil: For skin brightening

The anti-inflammatory properties of lavender oil make it able to brighten the skin. This is because it can lower skin irritation, discoloration, and redness and return the skin to its natural tone.

To use lavender oil for skincare:

Ingredients

2-3 drops of lavender oil

5 tablespoons aloe vera gel

Procedure

Mix lavender oil with aloe vera gel. Apply on the face with more concentration on the affected areas. Leave for 20 minutes then wash off. Do this once daily.

3. Rosehip oil: To fight wrinkles

The essential fatty acids and antioxidants in rosehip oil make it useful in cell regeneration. It cleanses the skin of lines and crow's feet.

To use rosehip oil for skincare

Ingredients

1 teaspoon rosehip oil

5 drops of lavender oil

3 teaspoons aloe vera

5 drops of lemon oil

Procedure

Combine all the ingredients in a glass bottle and shake thoroughly. Massage the mixture around your eyes before you sleep, every night. Rinse off in the morning.

4. Clary Sage oil: To heal wounds

Clary sage oil has antibacterial properties that make it potent against Staphylococcus aureus — the causative bacteria of pimples, carbuncle, and boils. Clary sage oil eliminates the bacteria from the affected area.

To use Clary Sage oil for wound healing

Ingredients

Clary Sage oil

Carrier oil (almond, olive, argan, coconut or jojoba oils)

Note: For every 10ml of carrier oil, use 2 drops of Clary sage oil.

Procedure

Using the right ratio, mix the essential oil with the chosen carrier oil. Rub on your face or area of concern. Leave it on till morning and then wash. Do this every day until the skin problem clears.

5. Geranium: To Help oily skin

Geranium oil is good for all skin types because it is not toxic, non-sensitizing and does not irritate the skin. Apart from that, it clears several skin problems like dermatitis, eczema and congested skin.

To use Geranium oil for skincare

Ingredients

3 drops of geranium oil

1 tablespoon of coconut oil

Procedure

Apply a mixture of the two oils on your face. Leave it on till morning. Do this every day or every alternate day.

6. Rosemary oil: For Face cleansing

Rosemary oil is an antioxidant that protects the skin from the harmful effects of free radicals. It is also anti-inflammatory and boosts circulation.

To use Rosemary oil for skincare

Ingredients

6 drops of Rosemary oil

1 tablespoon of aloe vera gel

Procedure

Make a face mask with the two ingredients. Massage it on your face for a while and allow it to sit. Wash it off after 15 - 20 minutes. Do this once daily.

7. Roman Chamomile: For clearing rashes

Skin rashes as a result of eczema, wounds, chickenpox, poison Ivy, diaper rashes and other skin conditions can be healed with Roman chamomile. This is because of the flavonoids and terpenoids it contains.

To use Roman chamomile for skincare

Ingredients

2 teaspoons Roman chamomile oil

¾ teaspoon water

2 ½ teaspoons almond oil

2 teaspoons lavender oil

8 tablespoons cornstarch

16 tablespoons baking soda

8 tablespoons Epsom salt

8 tablespoons citric acid

1 soap mold

Procedure

Blend all the ingredients into a paste. Pour the paste into the mold and press it. Allow the bath bomb to stand for 24 hours.

When it is ready, make a warm water bath and drop one bath bomb in it. Soak yourself inside to feel the healing benefits of the bath bomb on your skin. Do this twice or thrice every week.

8. Pomegranate oil: To stop photoaging

Pomegranate oil gets its antioxidant and anti-inflammatory properties from polyphenols. It lowers the effect of photoaging and inhibits the growth of skin cancer cells.

To use pomegranate oil for skincare

Ingredients

1 teaspoon pomegranate oil

10 drops of lavender oil

1 tablespoon jojoba oil (or any choice carrier oil)

5 drops of carrot seed oil

1 teaspoon rosehip oil

Procedure

Blend all the oils together and store in a container. Use it to massage your face before you sleep. Wash the mixture off the next day. Do this every day.

9. Frankincense Oil: To even out the skin

Frankincense oil is able to remove surgery scars, acne marks, stretch marks and other marks left by wounds and other things. This makes it able to calm irritated skin and even out the skin tone.

To use frankincense for skincare

Ingredients

4 drops of frankincense oil

1 tablespoon unrefined coconut oil

Procedure

Mix the frankincense oil with the coconut oil in a container. Store it in a cool, dry place. Wash your face then apply the mixture twice daily.

10. Lemon Oil: For Anti-aging

Lemon oil is able to lower oxidative stress on the skin and stop the free radicals from making the skin age.

To use lemon oil for skincare

Ingredients

20 drops of lemon oil

½ cup of safflower oil

Procedure

Mix the two oils into a bottle. Massage the mixture on your face and neck before retiring to bed. You can also use it on other body parts. Wash off in the morning. Do this once daily.

11. Sandalwood oil: For healing skin infections

Since ancient times, sandalwood has been used to treat skin conditions like boils, acne, rashes and other infections.

To use sandalwood for skincare

Ingredients

3-4 drops of sandalwood oil

1 tablespoon sweet almond oil

3-4 drops of lemon oil

Procedure

Mix the oils together. Use it to massage your face and neck. Allow it on for 30 minutes before you wash off. You can take as much time as you want though and do this once daily.

11. Ylang Ylang oil: For renewal of skin health

Ylang ylang oil contains antioxidants that help it to repair the lipids and proteins in the skin and keep them age free.

To use ylang ylang for skincare

Ingredients

2-3 drops of ylang ylang oil

Procedure

Mix the two oils together and then use it to massage your neck and face before you go to bed. Wash it off the next morning. Do this once daily.

12. Rose oil: For efficient absorption of skin nutrients

Rose oil is excellent at enhancing the skin's permeability to enable it to absorb the necessary nutrients and chemicals.

To use Rose oil for skincare

Ingredients

Rose oil (3 drops per 10ml of the product).

Any moisturizer or skin cream of your choice

Procedure

Mix the two ingredients based on the ratio. Apply on the skin regularly as part of your skincare routine.

13. Patchouli oil: For healing infections

Patchouli oil contains antiseptic properties that keep cuts and wounds on the skin safe from infection.

To use patchouli for skincare

Ingredients

15 drops of patchouli oil

¼ cup beeswax

10 drops of white fir oil

¼ cup of coconut oil

1/2 cup of olive oil

Procedure

Combine all the ingredients to form a skin cream. Use it on your hands and other body parts. Sleep with it and do it every alternate day.

15. Bergamot oil: For preventing bacterial growth

Bergamot oil is able to stop skin irritation and disinfect the skin by inhibiting the growth of pathogenic organisms that cause skin issues.

To use bergamot for skincare

Ingredients

20 drops of bergamot oil

Procedure

Prepare a warm bath. Add the essential oil to the water and add bath salts for extra benefits. Immerse yourself in the water and have a comforting bath. Do this thrice a week.

16. Cinnamon oil: To treat skin inflammation

Cinnamon oil contains a compound which treats inflammation and other conditions like rashes, dermatitis, eczema, itching, etc

To use cinnamon oil for skincare

Ingredients

10 drops of cinnamon oil

3 tablespoons honey

Procedure

Mix the oil and the honey. Rub the mixture on your face or the area of concern. Wash it off after 15-20 minutes. Do this once daily.

17. Cypress oil: As an antiseptic

Cypress oil is able to treat wounds, bruises and cuts faster than others and it is able to inhibit bacteria growth.

To use cypress oil for skincare

Ingredients

3-4 drops of cypress oil

1 teaspoon avocado oil

Procedure

Mix the two oils together. Rub on the affected area and allow it to sit for 30 minutes or more. Then wash it off. You can leave the mixture overnight and wash it the next day. Do it daily until the condition clears

18. Carrot Seed Oil: For natural sunscreen benefits

This oil provides vitamin A to your skin and makes it less sensitive to sun rays.

To use carrot seed oil for skincare

Ingredients

2 drops of carrot seed oil

1 tablespoon Shea butter

2 drops of frankincense oil

2 drops of lemon oil

Procedure

Blend everything together. Rub it on the face before you sleep. Wash it off the next day. Do this regularly.

19. Peppermint oil: For treating dandruff

The menthol in peppermint oil makes it effective in treating dandruff and boosting hair growth.

To use peppermint oil for skincare

Ingredients

10 drops of peppermint oil

4 tablespoons castor oil

2 tablespoons organic coconut oil

Procedure

Melt the coconut oil and mix it with the castor oil. Allow it to cool. Pour in the peppermint oil and store the mixture in a container, preferably bottle.

Use the mixture to massage your scalp and allow it to stay for the first 30 minutes. Wash off with a mild shampoo. Do this thrice or twice a week.

Chapter Eight

Carrier Oils

Carrier oils are the oils that are needed to dilute essential oils before using them topically. They help the skin to absorb the essential oils. Carrier oils are also used independently as ingredients for some lotions and skincare products.

Basically, carrier oils are vegetable oils gotten from the fat-containing part of the plant, like the kernels, nuts or seeds.

They are different from essential oils because they do not produce a strong scent and do not evaporate quickly. However, the carrier oils have a limited shelf life and can become rancid after a while. Carrier oils all have different characteristics and benefits. The color, shelf life, and aroma are all different.

These are some of the carrier oils that have been used together with essential oils in aromatherapy.

Almond Oil

Almond oil has several health uses. It is used to lower cholesterol, hydrate set skin, improve the cardiovascular system and stop inflammation. Using almond oil topically helps to calm and soften inflamed skin.

Almond oil is an antioxidizing agent that keeps the skin free from damage. It clears acne and also improves the health of the skin and hair.

Apricot Kernel

Apricot kernel is gotten from cold pressing the kernels of the apricot fruit. It is mostly used as a massage oil because it is gentle and light on the skin. People who practice traditional Chinese medicine use apricot kernel oil to heal ulcers and tumors. It improves skin health by removing acne, rejuvenating dry or inflamed skin, and healing skin conditions. It is also anti-inflammatory and stops swelling.

Arnica Oil

Since the 15th century, arnica oil has been favored for its therapeutic purposes. It has an anti-inflammatory compound named helenalin which makes it a suitable choice for use on the skin as a cream, salve, oil, liniment, and ointment. Arnica oil should be diluted before using it topically. Normally the arnica oil you'll buy in a store is already diluted but make sure you check the label thoroughly. Arnica oil provides relief for inflammation. It is useful in healing bruises, sprains, muscle pain, and some arthritis issues. It enhances hair growth and also has antibacterial properties.

Argan oil

Argan oil is obtained from the argan nut which is found in the Arab forest, in Morocco. It serves as a dietary supplement and a skin and hair booster. Argan oil is an important source of vitamins A and E. It is an antioxidant. On topical application, it releases it's anti-inflammatory properties, enhances the production of cells and serves as a moisturizer. It also exfoliates the skin and clears acne razor bumps, stretch marks, and burns.

Avocado oil

Avocado oil is extracted from the fruit of the avocado tree. It is gotten from the fleshy pulp of the fruit, unlike most edible oils that are extracted from the seeds of plants. Avocado oil contains healthy fat like essential fatty acids and oleic acid. The topical application of avocado oil will help to boost skin and hair health. It is anti-inflammatory and boosts nutrient absorption.

Coconut oil

Coconut is held in high esteem in India, the Philippines, the majority of Southeast Asia and other tropics. Coconut oil has a lot of health benefits and is widely used to make natural beauty products.

Coconut oil is capable of fighting bacteria and fungi, clears cellulite from the skin and improves the overall health of the skin and hair.

Evening Primrose oil

Primrose oil is gotten from a wildflower native to the Eastern and central North America. The oil is extracted through cold pressing of the seeds. This oil is able to alleviate PMS and treat some skin conditions and irritations. It helps to maintain hormone levels and enhance fertility.

Hemp oil

Hemp seed contains several ingredients that give the skin an all-natural vitamin boost. It has no THC (tetrahydrocannabinol) or the other psychoactive compounds that cannabis Sativa contains. Hemp oil has incredible amounts of omega fatty acids and protein which makes it an excellent choice for repairing the skin and removing acne and eczema. Hemp seed oil is an anti-inflammatory and antioxidant agent and helps in the removal of toxins from the body.

Jojoba oil

Jojoba oil is extracted from the seeds of *Simmondsia chinensis*. Jojoba oil is not an oil but a liquid plant wax that has been used traditionally as a cure for many ailments. It calms the skin and opens up hair follicles. Jojoba oil is a skin moisturizer and also an antibacterial and antifungal agent. It triggers the production of collagen and helps wound heal easily.

Olive oil

Olive trees have been around for a long time. Olive oil is extracted from the fruit of the olive tree and has high fatty acid content. It has antioxidant and anti-inflammatory properties. Apart from stopping oxidative damage, olive oil is also an antimicrobial agent. When using olive oil to dilute essential oils, it should be used in little amounts because it's fragrance could drown that of the essential oils. Olive oil helps the wound to heal fast and also heals UV damage.

Pomegranate oil

The pomegranate seed oil contains Anti-aging compounds. It contains bioflavonoids that act as sunscreen and sunblock. It has anti-inflammatory properties and helps to renew skin.

Rosehip oil

Rosehip oil is gotten from the seeds of the rose bushes that are common in Chile. It has potent antioxidants, essential fatty acids, and vitamins. The body easily absorbs rosehip oil because it is light on the skin. It acts as sunscreen and sun blocker.

Sea Buckthorn

Sea buckthorn oil is extracted from the berries and seeds of the plant. It contains several vitamins and minerals and it is used to prevent aging.

Shea butter

Although shea butter is not a carrier oil, it has several important properties that make it excellent for aromatherapy. Shea butter is a good moisturizer and has been an ingredient in many natural skincare products for years. It is an anti-inflammatory agent. It reduces eye wrinkles and acts as a sunscreen.

Chapter Nine

Some Conditions That Can Be Relieved with Essential Oils And Their Home Remedies

1. Acid Reflux

The essential oils needed to provide relief for acid reflux are:

Peppermint: It helps to loosen the gastrointestinal muscle making it easy for painful gas to gain passage.

Ginger: It calms the stomach and triggers it to release its contents in the small intestines.

Fennel: It maintains a proper pH level in the body.

Lemon: The compound present in the lemon peels known as D-Limonene helps to ease stomach pains and stop nausea.

How To Prepare An Acid Reflux Remedy

Prepare a beverage and add 1 drop of all the essential oils mentioned above. You can also add 1 teaspoon of coconut oil and honey to the oil blend and ingest it.

2. Acne

The essential oils that can provide relief from acne are:

Melaleuca: Provides antibacterial properties against skin dwelling bacteria responsible for acne.

Juniper Berry: Acts as an antibacterial but is soothing to the skin.

Holy Basil and Manuka: Possess antimicrobial properties that are good for combating acne.

Lavender: Prevents infection and has antibacterial and antifungal properties

To make acne face wash

Mix 20 drops of melaleuca, 1 tablespoon coconut oil, 2 capsules of probiotics, 1 tablespoon apple cider vinegar and 3 teaspoons honey.

Pour the mixture in a bottle and store. Keep it in a cool dry place.

3. ADD/ADHD

The essential oils that can provide relief for this condition are:

Cedarwood: Strengthens focus and mental clarity

Lavender: Induces relaxation and calmness.

Rosemary: Helps to improve memory and brain function.

How to make focus blend

Dilute 1 to 2 drops of vetiver with a carrier oil. Rub the oil blend behind the ears or on the wrists. For extra calmness and focus, add lavender and ylang ylang.

4. Addiction

Essential oils that can provide relief for this condition are:

Black Pepper and Peppermint: Soothes the discomfort caused by headache, nausea, and pain

Rosemary: Filled with mood-boosting compounds and relieves stress and anxiety

Lemon and Bergamot: Improve mood and build up energy

Lavender: Able to soothe the mind and improve mood.

How To make a soothing bath soak

Withdrawal symptoms and cravings can be reduced by preparing warm bathwater with 3 to 5 drops of lavender and Rosemary.

5. Adrenal Fatigue

Essential oils that can provide relief for this condition are:

Holy Basil: Lowers anxiety levels; helps balance the serum cortisol level.

Rosemary: Can reduce cortisol levels. Improves mood and memory.

Rose: Helps to reduce blood pressure and provides a soothing relaxation.

To make a warm adrenal compress

Mix 3 to 5 drops of either Rosemary or holy basil oil with a carrier oil. Rub the mixture directly over your kidney area. Lay a warm compress over it. You can also use the mixture on the soles of your feet.

6. Aging Skin

The essential oils that can provide relief for this condition include :

Ylang ylang: Capable of combating the growth of skin cancer cells and melanoma.

Lavender: Helps to avert oxidative stress that can cause early aging.

Frankincense: Helps to firm skin, clear acne spots and prevent wrinkles.

Sandalwood: Calms, cleanses and firms skin. Helps to lower inflammation

How to prepare anti-aging serum

Create a mixture of ¼ ounce of evening primrose oil, 10 drops of carrot seed oil, ¼ ounce of jojoba oil, 15 drops of vitamin E, ¼ ounce of pomegranate oil, and 20 drops of frankincense or lavender oil. Store the mixture in a dark glass bottle. Apply on your face and neck every morning and night.

7. Allergies

The essential oils that can provide relief for this condition include :

Eucalyptus: Assists in unclogging the lungs and sinuses

Ginger: Relieves allergy symptoms with anti-inflammatory properties

Peppermint: Clears sinuses and relieves scratchy throats.

Lemon: Purifies the body and helps in lymphatic drainage.

How to prepare a vapor rub

Get a glass jar and mix ½ cup of coconut oil, ¼cup of olive oil and ¼ cup of grated beeswax inside it. Fill a saucepan with water up to two inches and heat over medium-low heat. Heat the jar in the saucepan to melt the oils.

When it is slightly cool, add the 20 drops each of eucalyptus and peppermint. Store the mixture in a metal container and let it cool before application.

8. Alzheimer's disease

The essential oils that can provide relief for this condition include :

Bergamot: Enhances mood and soothes the body.

Frankincense: Improves the function of the immune system and provides immunity against harmful pathogens.

Lemon: Stops premature aging; boosts cell functions.

How to prepare a daily brain boost

Consume a daily mixture of 1 to 2 drops of lemon essential oil in a glass of water. Also, diffuse a mixture of Rosemary and lemon or apply topically to the back of your neck.

9. Anxiety

The essential oils that can provide relief for this condition include :

Roman Chamomile: Helps to relieve paranoia and calm aggression.

Lavender: Able to assist neurological issues like migraines and depression.

Frankincense: Helps to lower heart rate and blood pressure.

Vetiver: Enhances relaxation, soothes depression and insomnia.

How To prepare healing bath salts

Mix 1 cup of baking soda and 3 cups of Epsom salt. Prepare a warm water bath with 20 to 30 drops of lavender oil and 1 cup of the mixed ingredients. Immerse yourself in it for 20 to 30minutes.

10. Arthritis

The essential oils that can provide relief for this condition include :

Peppermint: Has muscle relaxing properties and is able to calm joint discomfort.

Wintergreen: Natural analgesic, helps to relieve pain and swelling.

Ginger: Lowers prostaglandin levels in the body.

Frankincense and turmeric: Lowers inflammation and boosts swelling

How to prepare detoxifying arthritis bath

Add 2 cups of Epsom salt, 20 drops of peppermint, and, 20 drops of lavender into a warm water bath. You can diffuse frankincense to give energy

11. Asthma

The essential oils that can provide relief for this condition include :

Eucalyptus: Assist in decongesting airways

Thyme: Maintains clean lung to improve respiratory function

Ginger: Clears mucus and stops inflammation of the respiratory system.

Peppermint: Clears the lungs and frees the bronchial passage.

How to prepare asthma remedy

Combine 1 teaspoon of coconut oil and add 2 drops each of thyme peppermint, ginger oil and eucalyptus. Apply directly on your chest and breathe deeply.

12. Back Pain

The essential oils that can provide relief for this condition include :

Turmeric: Helps to lower inflammation.

Frankincense: Enhances circulation and helps to lower inflammation caused by back pain.

Peppermint and wintergreen: Calms inflamed joints

Cypress: Boosts the repair of tissue and enhances circulation.

How to prepare a muscle rub

Mix ¼ cup of grated beeswax with ½ cup of coconut oil into a glass jar. Heat the jar in a saucepan with little water and medium-low heat until the contents dissolve. Put in 2 teaspoons of turmeric or cayenne powder.

After allowing it to cool, put in 15 drops each of lavender oil and peppermint oil. Mix properly and allow to set.

13. Bloating

The essential oils that can provide relief for this condition include :

Ginger and fennel: assists in calming bloating, indigestion and gassiness.

Juniper Berry: Helps the body to remove excess fluid.

Peppermint: Can help digestion by removing the gas in the GI tract.

Roman chamomile: Helps the gut to relax; it also helps stop inflammation.

How to prepare bloat-busting pre-meal routine

Before every meal, put in 1 drop of peppermint oil to a glass of water. You may also decide to consume a mixture of 1 to 2 drops each of ginger oil and peppermint oil diluted with coconut oil before meals.

14. Body Odor

The essential oils that can provide relief for this condition include :

Patchouli: Helps to naturally cover body odor.

Bergamot: Inhibits the growth of pathogens that cause body odor.

Lemongrass: Can be a natural deodorizer.

How to make a DIY deodorant

Combine ½ cup of baking soda and ½ cup of coconut oil in a bowl. Put in 40 to 60 drops of essential oils and store them in a deodorant container. Essential oils that can be used by women are lemon, Jasmine, sage, and lavender. The essential oils that can be used by men are cypress, bergamot, sandalwood, and Rosemary.

15. Bruising

The essential oils that can provide relief for this condition include :

Helichrysum: Soothes the skin, removes dark spot and stops pain.

Geranium: Boosts blood circulation

Lavender: Helps in cell regeneration and improves tissue health.

Frankincense and cypress: Helps to remove bruising marks.

How to make a bruise balm

Dilute 10 drops of helichrysum and 10 drops of geranium with ¼ cup of coconut oil. Spread the mixture directly on the bruise to improve healing and boost circulation.

16. Bug bites

The essential oils that can provide relief for this condition include :

Lemongrass: Possess high citral and geraniol content which helps to chase certain bugs like mosquitoes.

Citronella: Serves as a natural bug repellent

Holy Basil: Contains eugenol which gives it it's wound-healing abilities.

Lavender: Helps to speed up the healing process and produces a soothing feeling

How to make a bug spray

Prepare a spray bottle with ½ cup of apple cider vinegar, ½ cup of witch hazel and 40 drops of essential oils. Use a mixture of tea tree, citronella, lemongrass, and eucalyptus oils. Spray the mixture all over your body but avoid your mouth and eyes.

17. Burns

The essential oils that can provide relief for this condition include :

Peppermint: Can help burns by calming inflammation.

Lavender: Relieves burns naturally, helps to soothe and disinfect a site of inflammation.

Frankincense: Able to stop inflammation and scarring

Tea Tree and Manuka: This is able to lessen the risk of infection and calm the skin around the injury.

How to make a burn salve

Pour into a glass jar, 2 tablespoons of extra virgin oil, 20 drops of lavender oil and 2 ounces of raw honey. Rub the mixture directly on the burn or wound. Use a bandage to cover the injury site.

18. Cancer

The essential oils that can provide relief for this condition include :

Myrrh: Has anticancer properties that inhibit the growth of cancer cells.

Orange: Contains limonene that has chemo-preventive properties.

Turmeric: Is able to fight colon cancer, breast cancer, and leukemia because it contains turmerone.

How to prepare a triple cancer threat

Consume internally, 1 drop of myrrh, 2 drops of frankincense and 1 drop of turmeric oil thrice daily. You can also use the oils topically to provide support for an already existent cancer treatment plan.

19. Candida

The essential oils that can provide relief for this condition include :

Oregano: Is able to manifest it's antifungal, antiviral and antibacterial properties in the body.

Clove: Is known to be as effective as nystatin.

Cinnamon: Mostly efficient in combating pathogenic bacteria and fungi

Grapefruit: The d-limonene content helps to clear up the body's extra dampness.

How to prepare Candida remedy

Drink a smoothie with 1 drop of clove oil for two weeks. Do this under the supervision of a physician or nutritionist. You can also go on a sugar-free diet and eat mostly foods containing probiotic fermented foods, bone broth, organic meat, and cooked vegetables.

20. Chickenpox

The essential oils that can provide relief for this condition include :

Lavender: Helps in fast healing of scabs and blisters; clears skin itchiness and irritation.

Tea tree: Assists in reducing skin inflammation and combats pathogenic bacteria and infections.

Manuka: Calms the skin; antiviral properties help to clear most infections.

Roman chamomile: Penetrates the skin surface to boost skin health and stop irritation.

How to prepare pox ease

Dilute equal amounts of tea tree oil, lavender oil, oregano oil and lemon oil with coconut oil. Use a cotton swab to apply the mixture on your body thrice daily. Blend these oils with any oils that build the immune system and apply them on the soles of the feet and along the spine.

21. Common Cold

The essential oils that can provide relief for this condition include :

Lemon: Helps to clear colds and assists in lymphatic drainage

Thyme: Helps to reduce congestion, removes toxins from the body and fight infection; also clears congestion.

Ginger: Alleviates discomfort that is caused by infections and congestion.

Eucalyptus and peppermint: Helps In body cleansing

How to make a steam bath to relieve common cold

Prepare a hot water bath with 10 drops of peppermint oil and 10 drops of eucalyptus oil. Use a towel to cushion your head then inhale the steam deeply for 5 to 10 minutes.

22. Cough

The essential oils that can provide relief for this condition include :

Peppermint: Opens blocked airways and can stop sore throat pain.

Thyme: Boosts the immune system and reduces mucus.

Eucalyptus: Known to remove toxins and pathogens from the body.

Lemon and orange: Enhances the function of the immune system and induces lymphatic drainage.

How to prepare a cough syrup

Dilute 1 drop each of frankincense oil, lemon oil, Roman chamomile oil and peppermint oil with a spoonful of honey. Consume as needed.

23. Cuts and scrapes

The essential oils that can provide relief for this condition include :

Tea Tree and Manuka: Clear fungi and parasites.

Oregano: Has strong antimicrobial capabilities.

Cedarwood: Protects the body from bacteria.

Thyme: Helps to prevent infections on the skin and inside the body.

How to make a cut and scrape care

Use a clean towel and water to clean out the damaged area. Use hydrogen peroxide to remove any dirt present. Allow it to dry then spread 2 to 3 drops of essential oils with antibacterial properties on it and cover with a bandage. Change the bandage and add more oils every day to prevent infection until the cut is totally healed.

24. Diarrhea

The essential oils that can provide relief for this condition include :

Peppermint: Helps to calm the digestive system.

Roman chamomile: Relieves digestive distress and helps to manage emotional stress.

Ginger: It can enhance the function of the digestive system.

Turmeric: Improves the digestive system and lowers inflammation.

How to prepare a stomach ease

Dilute 2 to 3 drops each of peppermint oil, Roman chamomile oil and ginger oil with equal amounts of carrier oil. Apply the mixture on your abdomen. To get a more effective result, consume 1 to 2 drops of peppermint oil with honey for internal relief.

25. Ear infection

The essential oils that can provide relief for this condition include :

Basil: Combats bacteria and infections; commonly used for ear infections.

Manuka: Possesses antiviral properties which will help boost immunity and fight the cause of the ear infection

Tea Tree Oil: Has antibacterial and antiviral properties that make it useful in relieving ear infections.

How to prepare an ear ease

Mix 1 drop of frankincense oil with 1 drop basil oil. Apply the mixture behind the ears and on the soles of the best to hasten recovery time from ear infections. The mixture also helps to reduce swelling and pain. Before using the mixture on children, dilute with a carrier oil.

26. Eczema

The essential oils that can provide relief for this condition include :

Lavender: Boosts circulation in skin cells

Myrrh: Heals skin irritation; clears cracked or chapped skin

Geranium: Contains antibacterial compounds that relieve allergic reactions.

Manuka: Calms and helps fix damaged skin.

How to prepare eczema ease

Dilute 5 drops of geranium oil with 1 teaspoon of coconut oil. Apply the mixture on the affected area two times daily until the results are evident.

27. Flu

The essential oils that can provide relief for this condition include :

Thyme: Relieves infections of the chest and throat and has been proven to drain congestion.

Lemon: Has the ability to combat bacteria and viruses in the body and home.

Eucalyptus and peppermint: shown to rid the body of toxins and pathogens.

How to make a steam bath for flu

Pour a cup of boiling water into a bowl. Add 10 drops of peppermint essential oil or eucalyptus essential oil. Use a towel to cushion your head then inhale the steam deeply for 5 to 10 minutes.

28. Gingivitis (gum disease)

The essential oils that can provide relief for this condition include :

Cinnamon: Very effective in inhibiting bacteria that cause gum disease.

Clove: Helps to boost the remineralization of teeth and healthy gums.

Myrrh: Heals gums and diseases with anti-inflammatory content.

Tea Tree and Manuka: Prevents gingivitis with antibacterial properties.

How To prepare a natural gingivitis treatment

Mix 2 drops of any antibacterial essential oil like clove with 1 teaspoon of coconut oil. Sizzle the mixture in your mouth gently for 5 to 20 minutes to combat gingivitis.

29. Hair loss (alopecia)

The essential oils that can provide relief for this condition include :

Rosemary: Boost hair growth and fights against baldness, dandruff and slow greying.

Clary sage: Strengthens and firms hair follicles.

Lavender: Improves hair growth and lowers emotional stress.

Cedarwood: Assists in improving emotional well-being and thickening hair.

How to make Rosemary mint shampoo to prevent hair loss

Combine 10 tablespoons of baking soda, 6 ounces of aloe vera gel, 3 tablespoons of olive oil, 10 drops of peppermint oil and 20 drops of Rosemary oil. Store the mixture in a glass or plastic bottle.

30. Headaches

The essential oils that can provide relief for this condition include :

Lavender: Stabilizes mood, helps to lower muscle tension; shown to be an effective migraine remedy.

Peppermint: Helps circulation and lessens pain

Rosemary: Stimulates the body and reduces inflammation.

Eucalyptus: Opens congested nasal airways; relieves pressure on the sinus that leads to headaches.

How to prepare a headache ease

Dilute lavender oil, peppermint oil, and eucalyptus oil with a carrier oil. Apply the mixture to your temples, the nape of your neck and your chest. Then cup your hands over your nose and mouth and inhale deeply for some minutes before washing off.

31. Heartburn

The essential oils that can provide relief for this condition include :

Peppermint: Acts as a muscle relaxant and allows painful digestive gas to pass through.

Lemon: Assist in the excretion of digestive acids.

Fennel: Keeps the pH level balanced in the body, particularly in the stomach.

Ginger: Prevents the production of acid and stops ulcers.

How to prepare a heartburn quick fix

Make a mixture with 1 spoonful of honey, 1 drop each of lemon and peppermint oils, and 1 tablespoon of apple cider vinegar.

32. Hemorrhoids

The essential oils that can provide relief for this condition include:

Cypress: Helps to reduce swollen blood vessels; reduces inflammation.

Manuka: Helps in cooling the body and destroying bacteria and viruses.

Helichrysum: Stops inflammation and restores the blood vessels to a healthy state.

Frankincense: Helps to contract and firm tissues that hasten their regeneration.

How to prepare a hemorrhoid salve

Dilute 2 to 4 drops each of the helichrysum oil and cypress oil with a carrier oil. Use a cotton ball to spread it on the hemorrhoids. Do this every few hours as much as is needed to relieve pain.

33. Herpes

The essential oils that can provide relief for this condition include :

Myrrh: Contains antiseptic properties and helps to clean and treat cuts or wounds.

Manuka: Calms irritated skin, and reduces inflammation.

lavender: Nourishes and hydrates cracked or dry skin.

How to prepare lavender mint balm to relieve the condition

Heat 1 tablespoon of coconut oil, 1 tablespoon of beeswax, 2 tablespoons of Shea butter in a pot. Remove the heat and put in 7 drops of lavender oil and 7 drops of peppermint oil. Whisk the mixture properly and pour it into a tube or tins then allow it to cool.

34. Infection

The essential oils that can provide relief for this condition include :

Thyme: Has antiseptic properties that prevent infections inside the body and on the skin; also an antibacterial.

Tea Tree and Manuka: Has anti-parasitic and anti-fungal properties.

Cedarwood: Destroys bacteria in the body; protects the body from harmful toxins

Oregano: Shown to be a powerful antibiotic.

How to prepare an infection-fighting lotion

Squirt out some natural lotion and add 1 to 2 drops each of cedarwood oil, thyme oil, manuka oil, and tea tree oil. Mix well and rub on the sites of infection or the lymph nodes to combat internal infection. Also, consume oregano oil internally for two weeks.

35. Inflammation

The essential oils that can provide relief for this condition include :

Turmeric: Serves as an anti-inflammatory for the whole body including guts and joints.

Frankincense: Boosts circulation and reduces symptoms of muscle pain or joint pain.

Ginger: Helps to reduce inflammation with anti-inflammatory compounds like gingerol and zingiberene.

Patchouli: Stops internal inflammation and relieves conditions like gout and joints.

How To prepare anti-inflammatory rub/ pain reliever

Make a mixture of 10 drops of lavender oil, 10 drops of helichrysum oil and ½ cup of jojoba oil or coconut oil. Use the mixture to massage inflamed areas.

36. Insomnia

The essential oils that can provide relief for this condition include :

Roman chamomile: Provides a natural cure for anxiety and depression.

Lavender: Helps to keep the body relaxed; can also lower stress, anxiety, and uneasiness.

Ylang Ylang: Improves mood and relaxes the body.

Clary sage: Lowers inflammation and calms the body.

How to prepare a blend to induce sleep

Put lavender oil, Roman chamomile oil, and clary sage oil in a diffuser beside the bed at night, or use them to massage the back of your neck. You can also prepare a warm bath with Epsom salt to lower muscle pain and calm the body.

37. Irritable Bowel Syndrome

The essential oils that can provide relief for this condition include :

Fennel: Helps to induce body relaxation.

Ginger: Protects the internal issues with gastro-protective properties.

Peppermint: Helps to relieve IBS.

Roman Chamomile: Helps the body to relax and stops intestinal gas and bloating.

How to prepare IBS ease

Put 1 drop each of peppermint, ginger and fennel oils into some quantity of water thrice daily or mix the oils together and rub over the stomach twice daily.

38. Menopause

The essential oils that can provide relief for this condition include :

Roman chamomile: Helps to sedate the body, soothe the nerves and stop anxiety.

Clary sage: Relieves symptoms like hot flashes.

Thyme: Stimulates hormones that help to delay menopause.

Peppermint: Cools the body when experiencing hot flashes.

How to prepare a hot flash massage

Mix 5 drops of each of Roman chamomile oil, Clary sage oil and peppermint oil with 1 tablespoon of carrier oil. Massage the mixture on the body or use them in a warm bath.

Conclusion

I trust that you have gained much knowledge of essential oils from this book.

In truth, we owe the presence and use of essential oils in the modern world to previous civilizations. Indeed, most of the drugs we have now share the same herbal roots with essential oils. In reality, there are even more uses of essential oils than we have discovered.

Essential oils are a natural way of keeping body soul and mind healthy and you should grab the chance of using nature's gift to make your life better.